T0302793

What People a

Mindfulness Meditation & the Art of Reiki

Here is a book that explores the relationship between Reiki and the spiritual aspects that are the bedrock of its development. Steve Gooch takes the reader on a journey of personal development through the philosophy of Reiki and Buddhist tenets and practice. Foremost in these and a fundamental pillar of Buddhist practice (and other religious/spiritual traditions) is mindfulness meditation which has the aim of gaining insight into one's life, bringing the mind and body into harmony and assisting the path towards illumination or enlightenment.

Steve draws upon his many years of experience in Reiki and study of oriental healing/spiritual practice to lead the reader through key ideas and symbolic philosophy that is both original to Reiki and interpretational. This will inspire those new to mindfulness to step deeper into personal growth, practitioners of Buddhism to explore the human experience of body and mind through Reiki and practitioners of Reiki to discover the depth and breadth of Reiki as a spiritual activity.
Gordon Bell, senior Reiki Master

Steve Gooch's Mindfulness, Meditation, & the Art of Reiki guides the reader toward the deeper gifts and teachings held in holy silence at the heart of Reiki. He skilfully blends his knowledge of esoteric Buddhism with the system of Reiki to provide a framework for deepening your practice and experiencing Reiki as more than merely hands-on healing.
Nicholas Pearson, Reiki Master and author of *Foundations of Reiki Ryōhō*

Those yearning for a practical guide to access deeper levels of Reiki must read Steve's book! Through practical application

combined with spiritual practices, he shows us how powerful mindfulness meditation combined with symbols, mantras, breath, compassion, Reiki precepts and attunements or reiju significantly alter our perception of "what is Reiki." A detailed guide to awareness and wisdom awaits you.
Patricia Warren, senior Reiki and Buddho Master

I have been lucky and privileged to have been following Steve Gooch for over ten years on various platforms. His latest book is a fountain of knowledge and a reference for any Reiki practitioner who wants to deepen their own knowledge and understanding of the integrated universal relationship that Reiki has with all forms of spiritual teachings. Steve guides the reader and shows the importance of mindfulness in modern Reiki. The book is a definite must-have. It's a product of Steve's vast personal experience and diligent research.
Al Paton, Reiki Master

Mindfulness Meditation & the Art of Reiki

The Road to Liberation

Mindfulness Meditation & the Art of Reiki

The Road to Liberation

Steve Gooch

Winchester, UK
Washington, USA

JOHN HUNT PUBLISHING

First published by Ayni Books, 2022
Ayni Books is an imprint of John Hunt Publishing Ltd., No. 3 East Street, Alresford
Hampshire SO24 9EE, UK
office@jhpbooks.com
www.johnhuntpublishing.com
www.ayni-books.com

For distributor details and how to order please visit the 'Ordering' section on our website.

ISBN: 978 1 78904 889 6
978 1 78904 890 2 (ebook)
Library of Congress Control Number: 2021942980

A CIP catalogue record for this book is available from the British Library.

Design: Matthew Greenfield

UK: Printed and bound by CPI Group (UK) Ltd, Croydon, CR0 4YY
Printed in North America by CPI GPS partners

Contents

Meditations

Meditation on the Breath (Anapanasati)
Gassho Meditation
Meditating on the Symbols
Joshin Kokyu-Ho
Energy Gate Breathing
Six Point Meditation
The Body Scan
Metta Meditation
Open Awareness
Three Minute Breathing Space
Habit Releasers
On Duty, Off Duty

Also by Steve Gooch

Reiki Jin Kei Do
The Way of Compassion and Wisdom

978-1-90504-785-7 (Paperback)
978-1-78099-942-5 (e-book)

For Gordon and Dorothy Bell: my teachers. And for all those on a journey of self-discovery: the quest for love changes us.

Our lives become a creative expression of the transformation of energy, like ripples radiating out from the center of a pool.

Rob Preece – *The Psychology of Buddhist Tantra*

Preface

It was a hot, early summer's day in Cairo, Egypt, when I decided to embark on this book. To this day I am not sure why the urge to write it arose. I wasn't planning a book on Reiki. In fact, I was actively trying to avoid writing another Reiki book and had (and still have) a half-finished novel that was and is my main focus of attention, at least as far as my literary ambitions are concerned.

This current book began life as a short answer to a query by a student in Cairo, that then grew into a whole chapter. Realising that more could be said, I backtracked and wrote something to precede that chapter. I did the same again, writing what became Chapters 1, 2 and 3 in reverse order. At that point I realised that a whole book was emerging. I shed a tear for my novel and ploughed into Chapter 9 then 6, then 5 and 8 and 7, in that order. Eighteen months passed in the writing of it, spanning many months of tapping at my keyboard under the blazing heat of the Egyptian sun and finishing it off in the cold reality of the global coronavirus pandemic during lockdown in the UK.

This book marks a turning point in my understanding of the nature of the Reiki system and how it is so deeply interwoven with other spiritual practices, most notably with the practice of mindfulness meditation. More than this, however, on completing this current work it became apparent to me that a new door had been opened and that there are potentially other books, other avenues of exploration that can follow this one, most notably into a deeper investigation of Reiki's origins within esoteric Buddhism and Buddhist and Medical Qigong. Just how deep does the rabbit hole go? Only through plunging into it can that answer be found.

What I am certain of is that the current state of the literature on the subject has so far only scratched the surface. Reiki's journey out of the realms of New Age hokum into the world of being accepted as a serious spiritual practice will be a long one. It is going to take courage and a certain open awareness to all possibilities for Reiki to grow beyond where it is now. Most importantly it is going to take groundedness (the opposite of Reiki's recent populist trajectory).

It is my wish in presenting you with this book that two things can happen: that firstly you can find a new depth and meaning to your practice through bringing a grounded and philosophically meaningful orientation to the inclusion of meditation to it. Secondly, that now this book is complete, I can get back to finishing my novel.

Steve Gooch, Cairo, Egypt, January 2021.

Acknowledgments

There are several people to whom I would particularly like to offer my thanks for their help over the past year and a half as I worked on this book. There is no question that it would have suffered from a lack of confidence in its central message and focus had it not been for the ongoing support, encouragement and advice of my teachers, Gordon and Dorothy Bell, who diligently checked every chapter for me as it was completed. I am grateful for their continuing encouragement, twenty-four years after I first took my training with them. There are very few people in the world who I can genuinely, hand-on-heart, refer to as "Masters" of this discipline. Gordon and Dorothy unquestionably deserve this title. Their knowledge of the teachings along with their compassion, love and commitment to the practice have always been for me a shining example to follow on my own journey of self-discovery. This book would not have happened in anything like its current form without them.

A big thank you to Mark Hosak for his very useful comments on some of the finer points of Japanese culture and terminology and aspects of the history of Reiki as the book was almost ready to go to the publisher.

I am very grateful to Japanese artist Kazuko Komine for permission to use her illustrations of Seishi, Kannon and Dainichi Buddhas. Many thanks, Komine, and many blessings to you. A big thank you also to Hana El Ramly who posed for all of the photos for the meditation posture illustrations and to Heidi El Mahdy for her work in producing the illustrations for me.

I also want to thank Phil O'Neil for checking over the book as it was written and always being there on the other end of a Facebook message to supply me with much needed references when I was out of the country and unable to check them easily for myself, and for his continued friendship and support in so many ways. A special thank you goes to Taliya Tawfik for her precious and constant encouragement and support, for keeping me on track and always making me feel like I was doing something worthwhile when I felt like giving up. Your constant friendship is very precious to me, Taliya. A big thank you also for your photoshop skills when they were most needed! I would also like to give a special thank you to Nadine Reda who, in the sending of a short and fairly perfunctory WhatsApp message to me in April 2019, provided the catalyst for the book. This book's existence grew entirely out of that message which ended up being the pivot of its own chapter (Chapter 4). To Amal (Molly) El Masri for her friendship and enthusiasm and constant checking in on me to see how I was doing and then flooding me with her enthusiasm for this book. A big thanks also goes to Pat Warren, Nadine Reda, Maggie Ridge, Pete Grantham, Al Patton and Francesca Pinoni who kindly reviewed the book upon its completion and offered many suggestions for edits, tweaks and improvements which added substantially to the quality of the finished product.

I want to reserve an incredibly special thank you to my amazing friend, Amany Morgan, who has been a constant support throughout my journey with this book. All our chats and your patient encouragement over coffee at Beanos in Maadi, Cairo, made such a big difference to me over the months of writing, re-drafting and agonising over so many details of this book. Your friendship is such a profound blessing in my life, Amany.

I also want to thank my dad, Robert Gooch, who started me off on this journey via all of his books on Tibetan monks, pyramid energy, hypnosis, alien encounters and a whole range of other subjects that fired my imagination at a young age. Immersion in all these materials is what propelled me along my own path of self-discovery and creativity. And of course, I want to thank my mum, Pam Gooch, who taught me the true meaning of loving-kindness long before I ever encountered this as a Buddhist concept. I miss her deeply every single day of my life and carry her in my heart always. Finally, but by no means least, I must of course thank my wonderful kids, Marianne and Sam, who will forever be dazzling stars in the firmament of my life. I love you both so much.

Introduction

If you've been involved in the energy healing discipline of Reiki in recent years, you may have noticed that there seems to be a growing acceptance that its methods, teachings and philosophy are wrapped up with and underpinned by the practice of mindfulness meditation. More and more you find authors of books on Reiki exhorting their readers to engage with this powerful healing discipline from a place of mindfulness. Reiki Masters and national Reiki organisations are emphasising the need to be mindful when working with Reiki in a therapeutic context for the benefit of clients. But it hasn't always been this way. In fact, this is a relatively new phenomenon. During the 1980s and '90s and through to the early years of the millennium, no one seemed to care much about the concept of mindfulness within the practice of Reiki and it rarely got much of a mention. In those days everyone was still busy exulting over the miraculous and mind-blowing experience of the sensations of universal energy flaring and sparking like fireworks in the palms of their hands. Who could believe it? How was this happening? An air of excitement and incredulity pervaded the global Reiki community. Since then, things have quietened down a little and the understanding and approach to the discipline has become a bit steadier, more grown up and sober (at least in some quarters). The practice of Reiki is now a little less prone to being dressed up in the New Age accoutrements and spiritual flotsam and jetsam that it once was. As a consequence of this process of maturation, a much more sophisticated engagement with the practice, along with an understanding of the place of mindfulness meditation within the system has grown rapidly in the Reiki community. Mindfulness meditation is not a new addition to the system, however. Since its very early days, Reiki has been anchored deep into the bedrock of mindful awareness. Everything that we know of and understand about Reiki as a healing method is premised on the foundation of mindfulness. It's certainly true to say that without this mindfulness meditation practice, the system of Reiki would always be found skulking in the shadows of its true potential. If you want to drag Reiki out into the light and get a glimmer of what it really has to offer, you have to step back and take a look at it from a place of expansive awareness that is the consequence of a deeply committed engagement with the practice of mindfulness. From that place you would perhaps see that the great power behind all the razzmatazz and magic of Reiki energy is the stillness of the Absolute: the unmoving awareness within the infinite luminescence of the Universe. Within that awareness perhaps would come a distant glimmer of the potential radiance that the practice of Reiki can bring into one's life. This is the ordinary, mundane life that we all know and share. The *samsaric* life that Buddhists talk about: a life filled with un-satisfactoriness and suffering. If we could tap into that cosmic luminescence, we might change the trajectory of our lives and bring bliss and wonder back into our daily experience. But to do that, we must first knuckle down and commit to a meditation practice.

The fact is, Reiki never was, isn't now and should never be seen as just a simple hands-on healing therapy. When it is administered over a cosy chit-chat and a nice cup of tea in the back room of some nail bar, or to the sounds of Mongolian overtone chanting resonating in an incense filled evocation of a Bedouin tent (the New Age potpourri approach), the potential for the practice is being actively diminished. It can be so much more than this. Fortunately, Reiki is starting to be taken more seriously as a hands-on therapy and can now be found in various hospital and hospice environments in a number of Western countries. This is all excellent news, but we must be aware that it is far from being deeply embedded in these environments and we need to also be aware that in making a commitment to the view that Reiki is just a therapy, we are limiting the practice in quite profound and deleterious ways. This process of limitation is done, consciously and not-so consciously, so that it might somehow align in an uneasy truce with the dominant Cartesian model of health and healing that Western medicine demands of its allies. Going down that route has many potential benefits for the wellbeing of those in need of course and allows Reiki to contribute to the more expansive and holistic paradigm that is being cultivated by other alternative and complementary therapies. It most certainly should do this and, I feel, has a duty to do so. But in aligning itself in this way, the system of Reiki must be wary of losing its connection to its spiritual roots.

Beyond a therapeutic practice, Reiki has the potential to profoundly change the nature of one's experience of reality on all levels of being. The way to do that is to become aware. Deeply and profoundly aware. Of everything. All of the time. But just how do we do that in the context of Reiki? It seems that mindful awareness is largely assumed to be a skill that everyone already has when they first arrive at a Reiki class. This is not in any sense true. In fact, it's rarely taught at all and when it is, not properly. Even in the Reiki literature it is only cursorily mentioned and then dropped like a hot potato; after all, *everyone can already "do mindfulness," can't they?* it's reasoned. The fact of its existence within the system and the vague nod given in its general direction by all and sundry to attend to its cultivation has made zero impact on the evolution, understanding and outcomes of the Reiki system over the years. Worse, it is utterly ignored in any discussion of the philosophical underpinnings of the Reiki system, which in my humble opinion means that such discussion misses the heart of the system and diminishes it considerably.

Mindfulness meditation is a skill that needs to be taught and worked at. It is intrinsic to all styles and traditional expressions of Reiki around the world. Perhaps within Buddhist communities it can generally be assumed that everyone knows what mindfulness meditation is, if not from the perspective of a full-blown daily practice, then in a cursory way as a part of an inherited cultural and religious background. But Reiki has never existed solely within a Buddhist environment, not even within its original Japanese context. It has always been necessary, therefore, to explicitly teach mindfulness and encourage its cultivation. It's certainly important that we don't just assume that mindfulness is something that just "happens" automatically because we have learnt how to "do Reiki" (whatever that dreadful phrase means). Hopefully through the development and understanding of a mindfulness practice then yes, it does, in the end, just "happen." We can move from "doing mode" to "being mode" and so mindful awareness should simply arise. In the beginning, however, most of us need at least a little guidance on this topic. I remember teaching a Reiki class about twenty years ago and asking everyone in the class if they had any previous experience of practicing meditation. One answer stuck in my mind: "Oh yeah, I meditate sometimes. I really like to just lay on the beach with a glass of wine and a good book and really like, you know, chill, and catch some rays." Over the years I have been entertained a number of times with variations on the beach/wine/good book definition of meditation, including but not limited to: dancing/partying, taking drugs of various kinds, sleeping, and driving very fast around the Cairo ring road (!) (that's not to say that these things can't in fact be the subject of a mindfulness practice, just perhaps not the best choice as a means of developing a mindfulness practice). Then there is the ever popular "stopping your mind from thinking" approach (utterly impossible but an understandable misinterpretation of the nature of meditation). I learned right there and then that not only do many people attending Reiki classes not practice meditation at all, but that significant numbers of them have not the vaguest concept of what meditation is. It's most certainly not just chilling on the beach with a good book and a glass of wine or driving very fast around the Cairo ring road (although having been subjected to this by a number of Uber drivers, I can testify to the fact that you do in fact become intensely aware of utterly everything when traveling at speed on that road. But not in a good way!). Meditation can in fact be hard work. It can take focus, commitment, and persistence. Ideally, we want to eventually get to a place where meditation just happens spontaneously, revealing the true nature of who and what we are. If all of this isn't taught within a Reiki workshop, the gain from the system's practice is reduced quite considerably.

The lack of a mindfulness practice, or the lack of being taught mindfulness *properly* within the Reiki context means that practitioners are missing out on the many benefits that mindfulness has to offer. But also, they are missing out on the opportunity to bring a depth and quality to their engagement with Reiki as a therapeutic system.

In writing this book I wanted to spotlight Reiki's original formulation as a system of personal spiritual development. Almost every book ever written on the subject of Reiki focuses on it as a healing therapy. I felt it was time to redress that imbalance. Acknowledging the importance and, to my mind, primacy of the more personal and meditation-focused aspects of Reiki, we can find that our engagement with it as a therapeutic discipline is also enhanced considerably. In a sense this book is about squaring the circle of the direction given by Albert Einstein when he said

> *A human being is a part of the whole called by us 'Universe', a part limited in time and space. He experiences himself, his thoughts, and feelings, as something separated from the rest, a kind of optical delusion of his consciousness. This delusion is a kind of prison for us, restricting us to our personal desires and to affection for a few persons nearest to us. Our task must be to free ourselves from this*

> *prison by widening our circle of compassion to embrace all living creatures and the whole of nature in its beauty.* (Dyer, 2005)[1]

Our minds are conditioned by the world around us and so we view the world and everything and everyone in it, including ourselves, through multiple layers of conditioned perception. There is the layer of perception of our past experiences. There is the filter of our parents' influence, and of our schooling and that of our religion or lack of religion. There is also the filter of our culture and our moment in time, and then there is the filter of our projections and expectations of the future. So many layers of thoughts, emotions and judgments, obscuring and preventing us from seeing the world as it truly is; right here and right now. We have no idea from the perspective of the conditioned mind what reality really is. Our perception changes and shifts from moment to moment and so does the nature of our reality. Our conditioned version of reality is in a constant state of flux, shifting and weaving with our perception.

My hope with this book is that it will help in bringing some clarity of thought and of mind to the experience of working with Reiki and help to liberate it from the confines of the "healing therapy" box. The system can be much more than it currently is. Hopefully, through a better understanding of this Reiki method, a stripping away of some of the layers of obscuration that are impairing our understanding of the nature of reality and of ourselves as limited, dualistically orientated beings can take place. This is the bigger function of the system. If this book helps you on that journey of personal revelation and self-discovery, then it has done its job.

Throughout the book you will find scripts for the guided meditations that you can listen to and download at: www.omahhum.co/book-meditations. You do not have to have taken Reiki training to practice or benefit from these. However, the meditations described in Chapter 3 that are based on the

Reiki symbols, would potentially bring about more obvious and longer-lasting results for those who have received Reiki training first. If you have already taken training in the system, then please do try any or all of the meditations described in this book as a part of your regular Reiki routine. I am sure you will find them to be beneficial, not only as a part of a regular practice regime, but also within their own right as mindfulness meditations of scientifically validated and proven worth. Mindfulness, sometimes referred to as the "mind's gym" is increasingly being seen as a powerful health supportive discipline which is now being encouraged within formal health care settings across the world. Taking up the practice for its own sake is highly recommended but more so within the context of a well-rounded and considered Reiki practice.

All the meditations presented in this book can be accessed and downloaded here:
https://www.omahhum.co/book-meditations

Chapter 1

Getting to Grips with Meditation in the System of Reiki

From the 1930s onwards the Japanese art of Reiki has been known in the West as a powerful energy-based hands-on healing method. In practical terms a practitioner would place his or her hands either on or just off the body of a recipient and allow concentrated universal energy to flow. This would instigate a profound healing process for the recipient on all levels of being. That concept of Reiki started to change in the mid-1990s, however, with the publication of a book called *Reiki Fire*[1] by the German Reiki Master Frank Arjava Petter. Petter was the first Western Reiki Master to research the practice of Reiki in its homeland, and as a consequence of that research it rapidly became apparent that the system of Reiki was far more than just a hands-on healing method. As Reiki Master Taggart King noted:

> *Although Reiki is generally promoted in the West as a healing system, it seems that the original impetus for the development of Reiki was the personal benefits that would be experienced through the system to know one's true purpose in life and be content, to heal one-self and find one's spiritual path, and ultimately achieve satori.* (King, 2001)[2]

The primary function of the system then is as a powerful personal spiritual development practice. Reiki is as much about working on and developing yourself (if not more so) as it is about healing others through the laying on of hands, and there are various methods taught within the system to enable this to happen. Fortunately, as research into the origins of the

Reiki system goes on, we are slowly getting back to this much more meaningful and profound conceptualisation of Reiki as a spiritual practice rather than the one that sees it as no more than a simple energy healing method using the hands.

Reiki can therefore be seen in some senses as a dual system, having two distinct but symbiotically related orientations to practice which ultimately merge into one. If we look at how it is expressed within the Japanese traditions, even though they have a very strong emphasis on hands-on healing, there is an acknowledgement that Reiki should firstly be used to heal oneself. That is, it should be engaged with as a spiritual practice. Healing in its broadest sense is very much a spiritual practice with a focus on improving and perfecting oneself. It is a journey into deep healing. There is nothing wrong of course with viewing Reiki as just a hands-on healing method to use on other people, and we can personally receive many benefits from it in this form (it is a commonly known truism that we always receive a healing experience whenever we give someone else a healing session for instance). However, if we approach the practice first and foremost as a spiritual endeavor for ourselves (which naturally must encompass the practice of hands-on healing for others if we also receive a healing at the same time), we can receive many great benefits from it. It's really all about our orientation to the practice. It could be argued that the whole system of Reiki is entirely self-orientated and that the concept of treating "other" is really no more than a perceptual game, as there is on a macrocosmic level, no "other" to give a healing session to, and actually the more we work with the system in its conceptually pure form, the more we become aware of this truth. The concept of "other," of individuality, is a misnomer. We are all in fact simply emanations of the universal energy field, some would say of God; droplets temporarily breaking away from the ocean of oneness before we once more merge with it.

Central to a personal focus in the Reiki system is the practice of meditation. Reiki is as much about meditation as it is about working with spiritual energy in a healing context (personally, I would say that it is predominantly a meditation orientated practice and only secondly a hands-on healing method).

With the revelation in the West through the work of Petter and others that meditation is at the core of the system, almost immediately many Reiki Masters around the world started to add their own meditation practices to what they taught to "beef up" their classes in an attempt to modify their simple hands-on healing approach and turn it into a deeper, personal engagement with spirituality. In those days information about the true nature of Reiki was still thin on the ground, but things changed rapidly as more and more information began to surface.[3] Today, as the result of continuing research, we are in a much better position in our understanding of the original form of Reiki as a deep and powerful spiritual development practice. That understanding is continuing to evolve and develop as time goes by.

Across the world today there are many different expressions of the Reiki system. In the West there is the dominant hands-on healing form of Reiki that was originally taught from the 1930s onwards by a Japanese American woman called Mrs Hawayo Takata who had learned it in Japan in 1935. She became a Reiki Master in 1938 following a number of treatments for some health issues of her own. Then there are variations of Mrs Takata's Reiki that have bolted on various meditations and other practices, or incorporated the emerging techniques, methods and philosophy that sporadically flow out of Japan. There is also a plethora of New Age derivatives that have been developed over the years, largely in the West, but also in India and increasingly in the Middle East. In its home country of Japan there are many other expressions of the system that focus primarily on hands-on healing. These Japanese manifestations of the system tend to have some of the original spiritual methods and meditations as a solid foundation from which their hands-on healing work builds, unlike many of the Western approaches (which are in a constant state of "catch-up" with their Japanese counterparts). Then there are those methods, predominantly being advocated in the West by the likes of Reiki Master Frans Stiene,[4] that have as their primary focus the liberation from suffering of the practitioner. Whilst these approaches at their heart are also solidly orientated towards healing others, they very much build on the personal practice goal of moving towards the self-liberation from suffering of the practitioner, and not necessarily via the medium of hands-on healing. This is without a doubt the more sophisticated and more mature approach to Reiki (as I keep telling my students: if you want to heal the world, then focus on yourself and the world will follow).

At the core of all these approaches (except for some of the more ill-considered and bizarre New Age derivatives) is the fundamental requirement to bring a deep engagement with mindfulness meditation to your practice. It is implied in every aspect of the system and adds a profound richness to it. Mindfulness is the ability to be aware of what is going on right now: not reflecting on what has passed and not projecting forwards into what has yet to come. This is the bedrock and foundation of the entirety of the Reiki system in all of its numerous ways, facets and nuances of expression. As Taggart King has noted, mindfulness meditation was originally introduced at the start of a student's training in the system. It was later emphasized and developed further as the student progressed.[5]

Mindfulness

> *Mindfulness is the basic human ability to be fully present, aware of where we are and what we're doing, and not overly reactive or overwhelmed by what's going on around us.* (Mindfulness, 2014)[6]

Mindfulness is a meditation technique that was taught by the historical Buddha, 2,600 years ago and underpins all expressions of Buddhism around the world. It's a practice that can be undertaken whilst sitting, walking, standing, lying down or engaged in any daily activity. The ability to stay in the moment is a quality that is innate, but can be cultivated, developed and enhanced through proven techniques such as *anapanasati* (mindfulness of the breath). It's worth noting that in its classic form, as originally devised by the Buddha and expounded on in the *Satipatthana Sutta* (The Four Foundations of Mindfulness), mindfulness or *vipassana,* to give it its correct name, was very much a spiritual practice designed to lead the practitioner to the attainment of enlightenment. Accurately defining the concept of enlightenment, however, is as impossible as defining the concept of God (some would say that it's the same thing). As we have to start somewhere, we can use a broad-brush definition: we could say that enlightenment can be defined as the complete cessation of suffering and thus the removal of oneself from the cycle of rebirth. It is claimed that the Buddha's enlightenment came on the back of the practice of *anapanasati,* but mindfulness has other more mundane health benefits as well as the attainment of such lofty spiritual goals. The modern conception of mindfulness is stripped down and "lighter" than the original spiritual practice, with the goal perhaps being the easing of physical pain or to resolve mental and emotional trauma, or to boost one's ability to stay calm and centered in a stressful situation. Whether you are a spiritually focused *vipassana* meditator or a secularly minded mindfulness meditator, however, the practice is essentially the same.

Secular mindfulness is enjoying a global surge of interest of unprecedented proportions at the moment and is being used in a wide variety of healthcare settings around the world,[7] as well as in schools, prisons, hospitals and hospices for people with various ailments (mental, emotional and physical). Major corporations are using it to enhance employee wellbeing, reduce time off work and increase creativity and efficiency. It is even being used by the US marines to help them make more considered and rational decisions in the heat of battle.[8]

Like Reiki, then, mindfulness has a dual focus or quality: a secular, health and wellbeing orientated aspect, and a decidedly spiritual aspect. Of course, as has already been noted, they are ultimately and essentially the same thing.

Professor Mark Williams, the former director of the Oxford Mindfulness Centre in the UK said:

> *It's easy to stop noticing the world around us. It's also easy to lose touch with the way our bodies are feeling and to end up living 'in our heads' – caught up in our thoughts without stopping to notice how those thoughts are driving our emotions and behaviour... An important part of mindfulness is reconnecting with our bodies and the sensations they experience. This means waking up to the sights, sounds, smells and tastes of the present moment... Another important part of mindfulness is an awareness of our thoughts and feelings as they happen moment to moment.* (Williams, n.d.)[9]

When we practice Reiki, most of us are very much "living in our heads." It's almost as if our bodies are just vehicles for carrying our brains around. We ignore the presence of our physical body as our minds wander all over the place, projecting forwards into things that have not yet happened, or reflecting back on what has already passed. If we are in the process of giving a healing session, our flow of random thoughts might occasionally come momentarily to bear on the person under our hands, but it's probably not going to stay there for very long: *I hope they feel better after this, I feel really bad that they're having to suffer with all that pain/anxiety/depression/stress etc., I hope they can feel the energy, they might not believe anything has happened if they don't feel anything, What shall I cook for dinner tonight?* etc. We have all been there. Our minds are either forming their own arbitrary narrative structures; they're somewhere other than with what is happening right now, or are busy speculating, forming opinions, making judgments or otherwise engaged in a mental commentary based on the sensory data they are receiving. This gets mashed together with the storehouse of experiences, impressions and other mental events that the mind has filed away to form new lenses through which to view the world, and none of this is helpful to us or beneficial to the person receiving the healing session. We need to stop thinking about the past and the future and refrain from worrying and speculating and judging and pondering on intangible concepts. We need to get out of our heads and into our bodies and focus on the *now* from a perspective of pure, clear awareness. And we should avoid allowing our minds to get involved in the healing session that is going on under our hands. I will come back to this later.

> *There are many good reasons for practicing mindfulness of body. We live in a society that exalts thinking – our education system prioritises academic learning, and most people are trained when they're young to identify with thought. Even the English word 'mindfulness' makes our subject sound like a quality of thinking. Whereas actually, mindfulness brings us down from our heads and into our whole bodies. Ask someone from Tibet where their mind is and they may point to their chest – the word for mind and heart in Tibetan, and many other eastern languages, is the same. When we practise mindfulness, we're recalibrating our centre downwards – as such, the practice might better be described as 'heartfulness', or even 'bodyfulness'.* (Halliwell, 2015)[10]

So, even though when we think of mindfulness, or awareness, we tend to think of what is going on in our head, it is more accurate to think about what is going on in the whole body. Consciousness is not just located in the head; it is everywhere in the human being and we should keep this in mind when we work with mindfulness as a meditation practice. We need to sink our awareness into the abdominal area: down into our core where we feel our breath as infants, centered on the umbilical cord. As we shall see later, this is critical to our exploration of what are called "the three elixir fields."

All of this is of significance to us as practitioners of Reiki. Whether we are engaged in giving someone a healing session or whether we are working on our self, mindfulness should be the primary practice. Having our minds wandering all over the place is not conducive to progress in the system of Reiki, and it certainly isn't conducive to an effective or meaningful healing session for someone else. But more than this, a well cultivated ability to be aware, to engage in our "Being Mode" rather than our "Doing Mode" really does have a profound impact on our ability to get the most out of the system. The "Doing Mode" is the mind's ability to solve problems: getting us from where we are now, to where we want to be; breaking down information and analysing it to see if it can find a solution. We use this mode for everything from designing a new skyscraper, to creating a work schedule. As Vidyamala Burch and Danny Penman made clear in their wonderful book *Mindfulness for Health*: "Being mode is not bigger or worse than Doing mode, just different. It's bigger than thinking. Kinder than thinking. And can often be wiser than thinking too" (Burch and Penman, 2013). As Reiki practitioners, this is where our heads should be when engaging with this deeply profound system. We need to be developing our mind of wisdom (insight) and not just our hearts of compassion, and we need to stop this:

2.00pm: *My client arrives at the door and rings the bell... I quickly swig back the last of my coffee and head for the door... I hope she doesn't talk much... I need to go out and get some material for the fancy-dress costumes for the kids right after this... I wonder where Sally got that material for her kids? I should ask her... that's if she's talking to me... it's not my fault the dog dug up her lawn... she should have kept the gate locked... besides she deserved it for the mess her cat made of my flower baskets that time when we had the BBQ...*

2.05pm: *My client comes in and smiles... oh, I like her skirt... I wonder where she got it from. That would match the new top I got last week... I could have spent a fortune in the sales... I will miss that shop... I wonder what will open there next... Maybe they'll knock it down like they did with the cinema... it's ages since I went and saw a good movie...*

2.10pm: *Client climbs on to the bed... please don't break, please don't break... thank God... I smile... I do my dedication and put my hands on her head... what was I thinking? Lovely skirt... But with my figure? I really should try that new diet from the magazine... it sounds really good... but I'm not sure I can quit chocolate altogether... Mike's a pig; always hiding the chocolate where I can't find it... I wonder what time he gets home today...*

2.15pm: *Move hands... God I am bored with this today... I don't want to do this... what's that perfume she has on? I really like that... I must ask her... I hope she doesn't fall asleep... I need a quick getaway when this is over... I might even have time to meet Sally for a coffee... if she's talking to me... she can be so childish sometimes... no wonder her husband had an affair... etc., etc.*

It is not always easy to stay in the moment; to stay present. Most of us, in our first tentative efforts with mindfulness, would relate very well to Vessantara's description of his experiences of learning meditation when he said in *The Art of Meditation: The Breath*:

> *I often struggled to find the breath for more than a few seconds at a time. I felt like a shipwreck survivor clinging to a spar – the breath – while great waves of thought crashed over me. Their tremendous pull frequently dragged me under. I would surface seconds or minutes later and then swim back to the distant spar, get a loose grip on it, and then be washed away by yet more feelings and ideas.* (Vessantara, 2005)[11]

When we can put the time and effort in to train ourselves to use the breath as a dynamic anchor for our awareness, we will eventually have something to pin our consciousness to. It is worth noting the words of the Buddha in relation to this, however, when he made it clear that in the practice of mindfulness, we should attempt to have mindfulness of the body *within* the body and mindfulness of the breath *within* the breath. That is, we are trying to fully become the body or the breath, rather than holding on to an artificial split between our awareness and the object of our awareness. When we can do this, it reveals the mind's Doing mode in action. We can step back from our thoughts and look at them rather than from them. We gain the ability to experience the world directly rather than through the filter of our suffering and our sensory attachments, which cause so much of that suffering. This is the Being mode. We realise that as we bring our awareness to the breath, when we immerse ourselves fully in the experience of the breath, we can only take a breath for this moment. It's impossible to take a breath for the past or the future. These breaths are no more than concepts, not experiences.

As we start to appreciate the transitory nature of our breath as it rises and falls, and as we see the passage of our thoughts across the stillness of our minds, we begin to appreciate that nothing is fixed or permanent and that there is only this moment. And that likewise, we ourselves are transitory in nature. There is nothing fixed and permanent about us. The suffering that we and others experience is because of the illusion of permanence and our attachment to it.

This "being" that we consider to be "I" is not one solid permanent being, but consists of body, mind and breath. Breath and the body are matter, and awareness of the breath is mind. As we practice and become aware of these interlinked aspects of our being and their state of impermanence, the concept of "I" starts to break apart.

As Shunryū Suzuki noted in *Zen Mind, Beginners Mind*:

> *If you think, 'I breath,' the 'I' is extra. There is no you to say 'I'. What we call 'I' is just a swinging door which moves when we inhale and when we exhale. It just moves; that is all. When your mind is pure and calm enough to follow this movement, there is nothing: no 'I', no world, no mind nor body: just a swinging door.*[12]

We are, then, simply processes in a constant state of renewal: coming into being and passing away. When we practice mindfulness and when we practice Reiki, all that exists is the movement of the breath and we are aware of this movement. When we are aware of this, we are aware of our True Nature, our universal self, and we can become conscious of merging back into the ocean of oneness (which in truth, we had never left in the first place).

Meditation Posture

So how do we practice mindfulness meditation? Firstly, we need to consider our posture. Given that Reiki is a Japanese practice, it might be appropriate to sit in *seiza* (which means "correct sitting"). This posture, however, designed so that samurai can get up quickly during a fight, can be extremely uncomfortable for those not used to it, and given that it has only existed in Japanese culture for around 200 years can easily be discarded for less painful postures. If you wish to try sitting in *seiza*, however, this is how:

Kneel with your buttocks resting on your heels. Your back should be straight, and your hands should be folded in your lap. Men can have their legs slightly apart. If you find that sitting in *seiza* for any length of time is uncomfortable (and you probably will) you can always try using a meditation cushion with your legs either side of it. In Zen meditation (*zazen*) a square pillow called a *zabutan* upon which sits a round pillow called a *zafu* is used, but any comfortable cushion will do. Or you can use a meditation stool (sometimes referred to as a *seiza* bench) which is very stable but without all the discomfort associated with crushing your ankles with your full body weight. It should be noted that the *seiza* posture is in fact very stable and according to Karlfried Durckheim one that "is in accord with nature." He goes on to say, "Why does a five-story pagoda not collapse? Because it keeps its physical balance. If one sits in the seiza posture one does not topple over no matter from which side one may be pushed."[13]

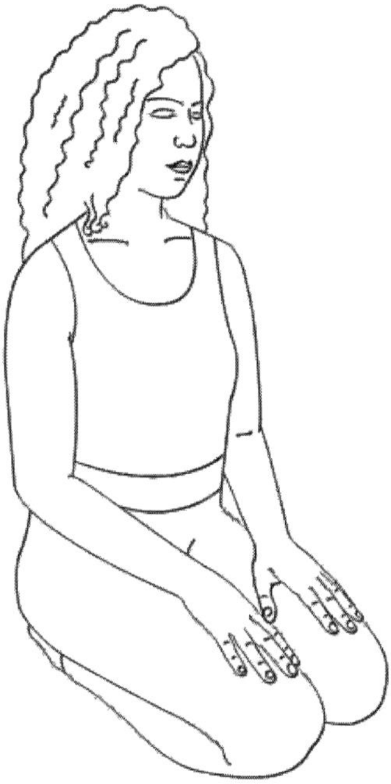

If *seiza* doesn't work for you, you could try sitting cross-legged in a lotus or half-lotus posture. If that is also uncomfortable, you could sit on a chair. The lotus is a traditional meditation posture and the one favored by Gautama Buddha when he achieved enlightenment under the Bodhi tree two and a half thousand years ago. If you also find that difficult, you could try sitting in a half lotus over an extended period, to see if your leg muscles will loosen up so that you can get into a full lotus more easily. The main difference between the half and full lotus is that the knees are both touching the floor in the full lotus, which gives a much more stable posture. If your knees are floating in the air higher than your hips, you are unstable. Stability in meditation (both body and mind) is a critical element.

I generally use a meditation stool or sit on a chair to meditate but let's assume you are significantly more flexible than I am, and you can get into a full lotus posture. You should have your left foot on your right thigh and your right foot on your left thigh. In traditional teachings this posture is considered to represent the oneness of duality. It doesn't represent oneness or duality individually, but both at the same time. It's the same with the body and the mind. They are obviously two very different things but simultaneously they are also fully integrated elements that come together to form one being. You should keep your spine straight, resting in its natural curve, with your shoulders relaxed but in line with your ears. Also pull your chin in so that it is not tilting upwards or downwards. Allow your hands to form the cosmic *mudra* (*hokkai-join* in Japanese). The left hand should be on top of the right hand, with the middle joints of the middle fingers touching (some say that you should have the dominant hand as the lower hand with the other hand cradled in it. I have tried both ways and find little difference). Touch your thumbs together so that they form an oval shape. Your hands should be close to your body, near your navel. You may like to place a cushion on your lap to take the weight of your hands and arms.

Your arms should not be too close to your body, however. Allow a little space under each arm pit and sit with dignity, as if you are holding up the sky with your head. Your neck should be soft and your shoulders sinking downwards (but not slumped forwards). Place your tongue to the roof of your mouth, just behind your teeth and either close your eyes or have them half open with your gaze a few feet ahead. When you hold this perfectly balanced and stable posture, your mind is much more likely to assume a balanced and stable state. Mental stability and focused awareness are a lot more difficult when done slouching against the back of a chair or a wall as seems to be the practice in so many workshops these days.

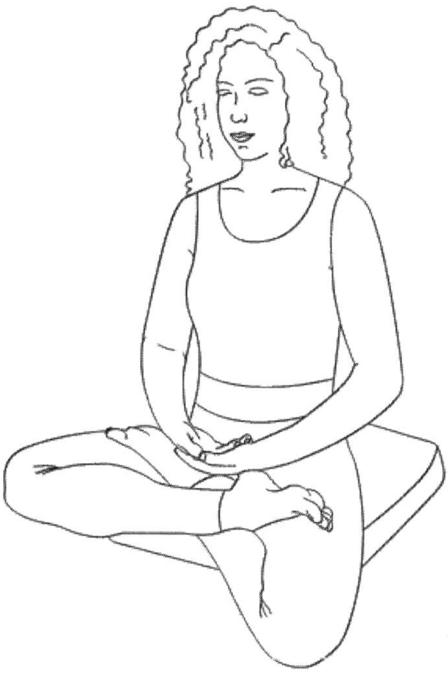

If you are using a chair, sit independent of its back. To begin with you might have some lower back pain. Check that your knees are not higher than your hips. If this is the case, you will overwork your lower back and cause discomfort. Place a firm cushion on the chair first if necessary. If you still have pain in this area, it might be because most of us rarely exercise our lower backs due to sitting for long periods. Normally we lean against the back of the chair, allowing our lower back muscles to rest. When we sit independent of the chair back, these muscles must start working. It is worth just sitting through the discomfort for a period until your back muscles get used to working properly. Of course, if you have lower back problems or other physical restrictions that mean you can't assume a good meditation posture easily, you should use some sort of support. It is always best to be fully independent of any physical supports as much as you can, however. Our bodies should be physically independent, and our minds should be mentally independent.

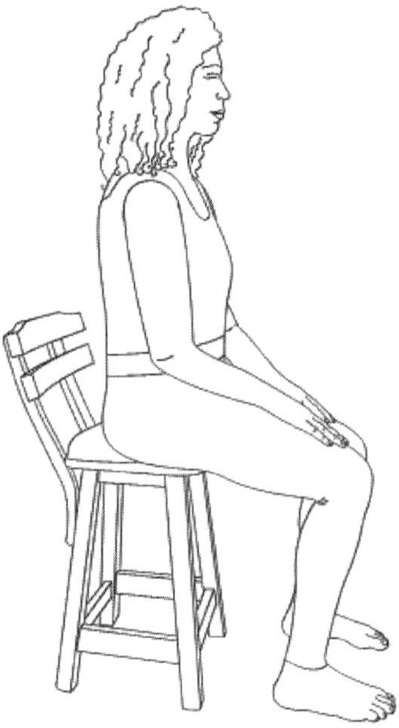

It is also possible to simply lie down to meditate and you may find this to be of great benefit if you struggle with sitting for any length of time. The Buddha described four types of meditation posture; from the most inactive to the most active: lying down, sitting, standing and walking. If you wish to lie down, we could look to Zen for some help in describing the classic postures. A word of warning: it is best not to lie on your bed as we have so programmed our minds that lying on the bed means it's time to sleep, that it is extremely difficult to do so and stay focused and alert.

There are two lying down postures favored in the Japanese Zen schools. Here is the first:

Lie on your back on the floor, or if you wish, on a yoga mat or rug. Extend and splay your legs with your feet out to the side. Your hands should be either folded onto your belly (*hara*) or placed down beside your body, but a little way from it, with the palms facing upwards. If you have lower back problems, it's okay to place a cushion or bolster under your knees with your feet flat on the floor. Your knees should be pointed towards the ceiling. If you wish to place a pillow under your head also, this is fine. Lengthen and straighten your back without straining it.

The second method is as follows:

Lie on your side – traditionally this would be the right side. Bend your knees slightly and have one leg on top of the other. Your lower arm should be stretched upwards and away from the body so that the head can rest on it. The other arm can be resting down the side of the body. If you wish you can bend it at the elbow so that the hand or fist is touching the floor. Again, if you wish to have a pillow under your head, this is fine and you can also place a bolster, cushion or rolled up towel under your waist for support. Lengthen the spine as you did in the previous prone posture without overdoing it. In both of these lying down postures, you should be relaxed with no undue strain.

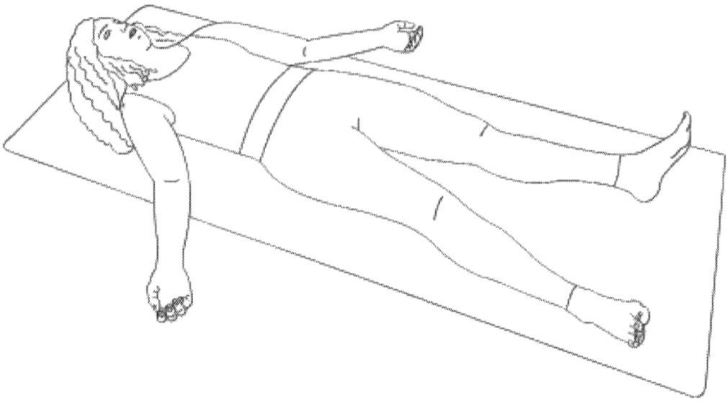

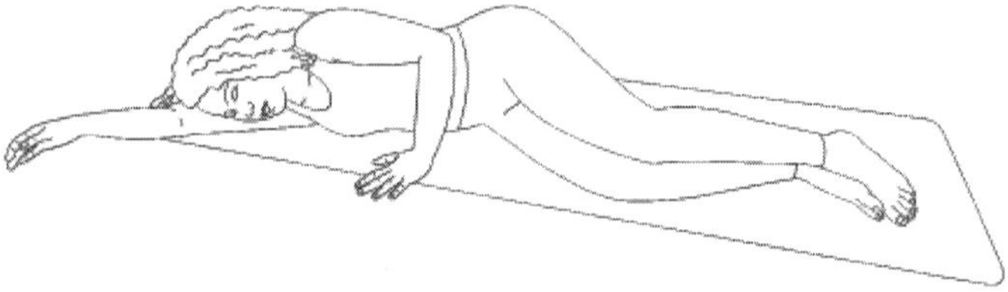

In establishing a successful meditation practice, you must ultimately find what works for you. I have given you some postures that you might like to try. Perhaps you could experiment and try out different approaches. This is especially true if you suffer from some physical impairment or if you are bed-ridden or have some other issues that prevent you assuming a traditional meditation posture. If none of these traditional approaches are possible, it's perfectly acceptable to get creative and find your own way with this. The important requirements of a good posture are that you are stable, comfortable and alert.

Mental Equipoise

Do you play tranquil New Age music or recordings of the sounds of nature when you sit to meditate? So many of us do this and mostly because others have introduced us to it, or we've attended workshops where this is part of the "spiritual baggage" used to create a certain type of ambience. It has become an expectation within the New Age/alternative healing community. The playing of such music or sounds as an accompaniment to a meditation practice is never questioned. Perhaps it should be. Just as our body should be independent of external support and completely stable, so should our mind. When did you see video footage on TV of monks with their headphones on listening to their favorite tunes while they meditated? Of course, you didn't. When you are using an external support such as music, your mind can become reliant on it and influenced by it. When the music gets sad, your mood can change. When the music gets happy, you can get happy. This is not meditation. This is relaxation. One of the things that mindfulness practice does is reframe your relationship with these types of sensory input. Give yourself a fighting chance with your practice and turn the music off. It really isn't helping you.

We need to learn to work with the mind during meditation, rather than against it. As we all know, our normal day to day is made up of thousands of thoughts drifting (and sometimes rampaging) across our minds. We are reflecting on the past or projecting into the future, and rarely spending time in the only reality that exists: *now.* And when we sit to meditate for the first time, we somehow expect this normal mental activity to cease entirely and our minds to just be still and empty: a vast open void of nothingness, of perfect clarity and intense bliss. Of course, this is about as far from the true experience of most meditators as you can get. When we sit our minds continue with their normal activity: trying to think about lunch, wondering if the neighbor is having an affair, planning the finances for next year's holiday etc. And when this happens, we tend to feel frustrated and let down because we can't make our minds stop thinking. However hard we try we simply can't do it. Why is this? Because the mind is designed to think, and it is very good at it and has had a lifetime of experience of doing just that. When we begin a meditation practice, such as *anapanasati*, it's very important to remember that our job is not to stop the mind from thinking but to simply be aware. We cannot force stillness upon the mind. All we can do is watch the breath, which will tend to have a naturally calming effect on the mind. In its own time, the mind will gently slow down and the thoughts will arise less and less often. Even for the most experienced of meditators, however, thoughts arise and roam across their minds from time to time. One method that we can use to help settle our minds at the start, and at any point during a meditation, is to sink our consciousness down into the belly or *hara*. Anchor your attention there and feel the movement of the belly. You might want to slow your breathing a little or take a few deeper than usual breaths before allowing it to return to normal once more. Focus on your out breath and allow your body and mind to settle. Placing your attention here gives a sense of being anchored and helps to draw energy down from the head, thus slowing the rampage of thoughts that are competing for your attention and taking you away from the breath. Conversely if you are feeling tired and your eyelids are heavy and you keep drifting towards sleep, you can take a few short, shallow breaths high into your chest and focus on your in breath. This will help to energise you. So, to be calm; go deep down into the core of the body, and to energise; go high up in the body.

When we can become aware, then we are doing the job of meditation. Sometimes if a thought arises, we can get sucked into the mental commentary that arises with it. This can go on for some minutes before we realise that we are supposed to be watching our breath. When we do finally become aware of our mind's wandering, we can simply bring our awareness back to the breath. It's important at times like this not to get frustrated with ourselves and think that we are failing in the meditation. In fact, we are succeeding. We are doing exactly what we sat down to meditate for: to become aware. Each time we catch our mind wandering, this is a moment of awareness, of success. Becoming aware of your wandering mind is the first sign of mindfulness taking root; simply bring the mind back to the focus and continue, and if we must do this a hundred times over, it's okay. That is a hundred moments of success right there. With practice we find that these moments of awareness happen more frequently, and so they start to join into a seamless flow of awareness.

It is also important to have patience with ourselves. So many times, I have heard from students in Reiki classes that they can't meditate. "It's just me," they say. Everyone else in the world, they are sure, can meditate just fine, except for them. They consider themselves as being somehow unique in their inability to meditate. When Shakespeare first picked up a pen, or Jimi Hendrix first picked up a guitar, or Picasso first picked up a paint brush, did they give up in despair a week after their first feeble attempts? Of course not. To master anything, you must dedicate yourself to it. You need to practice daily for long periods of time, over and over again. There is one difference, however, between meditation and these other pursuits. To be a writer, a musician or an artist, you must have some sort of definite goal in mind, a level of achievement or success which you wish to attain. Meditation isn't like that. In meditation, we simply sit, to sit. We don't set an outcome or goal or try to attain something. We sit, to sit. You cannot fail at meditation.

Shunryū Suzuki, the great Zen teacher said that when we sit to meditate with the intention of doing something special such as achieving enlightenment, we are doing nothing at all. When we sit, just to sit, then we are doing something special. This is when we start to become and embody our True Nature.[14]

Meditation on the Breath

Having understood the need for a good physical and mental posture, what next? Let's go through a basic *anapanasati,* or mindfulness of breathing practice.

Let us begin by establishing our meditation posture and placing our hands in the form of the "cosmic mudra," or if you wish, you can simply place your hands palms down on your legs. Then mentally run your mind over your body checking your posture. Make sure that your spine is straight, but not over-extended. Your spine should be resting in a natural S-shaped curve. If you are using a chair, make sure that you are not leaning against the back of it unless you need the extra support, and that your feet are planted firmly on the floor. Make sure that your body is natural and relaxed. There should be no sense of straining.

Check that your shoulders are not tense. As you breathe out, consciously allow any tension in the shoulders to slip away. You should feel a sense of openness in the chest. Check that your head is balanced gently, imagining that you are supporting the sky with the crown of your head. Now close your eyes or half close your eyes and let your gaze gently fall a few feet in front of you. There should be a sense of quiet dignity about your posture.

Bring your attention to your breath. Notice the breath as it goes in and out. Try to really tune into it. Notice where it first hits the point just below the nostrils before it enters the body. Perhaps you can feel a cool sensation as the air passes through the nostrils on its way to the lungs. Feel the rise and fall of the belly with each breath as the diaphragm broadens and flattens and then rises back up underneath the ribs. Can you be aware of your chest expanding and contracting?

Try not to change the breath. You are not "doing" something with the breath, you are just observing it. Allow the breath to do whatever it needs to do. Just gently follow it in and out. If your mind wanders, this is okay. This is the natural process of the conditioned mind. When you notice that it has wandered, just gently bring it back to the breath. If you need to do this a hundred times, it's okay. You are not failing when your mind wanders. Every time you notice that your mind has wandered, this is a moment of success, of awareness. Have compassion for yourself.

Now go a little more deeply into your body. Where are you feeling your breath the most? Can you feel the rise and fall of the body with each breath, like an ocean swell? Feel the natural movement of the breath and the body.

Stay with this process for two or three minutes: watching the breath going in and out. We are using the breath as an anchor for the mind. Each time the mind wanders, we anchor it back on the breath. In order to notice that the mind has wandered, there must be something bigger than the mind that has a wider perspective. This wider perspective is awareness. It is much easier to handle the mind when it wanders in the wide open space of awareness. Just like the sky stays still and serene as clouds gather and pass across it and then dissolve into its vast emptiness, so your thoughts will gather, roam across the vastness of your awareness and then dissolve into nothingness.

Now just gently bring your awareness to the weight of your body sitting on the cushion, the floor or the chair. Feel the weight of your hands and your arms resting in your lap. Gently extend your awareness back out into the room that you are in, becoming aware of the surroundings. Take a few deep breaths, connect with your feet and open your eyes.

Through practicing a basic mindfulness meditation such as this, we are equipping ourselves with the necessary tools to bring to life one of the most basic components of the Reiki system: The Reiki Precepts. Mindfulness is the bedrock of the Precepts. If you don't practice mindfulness, you stand little chance of bringing them to life. They are not just hollow refrains but something that needs to be lived in each moment of our lives.

Chapter 2

Bringing Mindfulness to the Reiki Precepts

The Reiki Precepts, often marginalised or forgotten about by so many students at the end of a Reiki class, are the central pillar of the personal development system created by Mikao Usui, the founder of Reiki.[1] The precise origins of the Precepts are not known, but it is generally assumed that they were based on a similar set of Principles as set out in the book *Kenzen no Genri* by Dr Suzuki Bizan.[2] It's also possible that they were based on ninth-century Buddhist precepts.

There are two known versions of Usui's Reiki Precepts: one version, it's claimed, was brushed by Mikao Usui himself, and the other is carved into his memorial stone. There are only slight variations between them. These Precepts are the guiding principles of the whole of the Reiki system and can be found in various forms in all schools of Reiki around the world.

There are many extant translations of the Reiki Precepts (or *Gokai* in Japanese). All of them are approximations of the original Precepts that were given by Usui and all say essentially the same thing. Given that they were originally expressed in Japanese, however, there will always be distortions due to transliteration when presented in other languages. The following version, which serves us better than most, is from Frans Stiene's *The Inner Heart of Reiki: Rediscovering Your True Self*[3]:

The esoteric teachings to invite blessings
The spiritual medicine of having strayed from universal truth:

Today only
Do not anger
Do not worry

Be grateful
Practice this diligently
Be kind to yourself and others

Perform Gassho in the morning and evening
Be mindful about this in your heart/mind
Chant with your mouth
Improve your heart/mind and body

Usui's teachings (dharma) to cure and heal one's True Self
The founder Usui Mikao
(Stiene, 2015)[4]

I would like to focus on some important elements of the Precepts that often get glossed over that relate to the practice of mindfulness. The very first line; "The esoteric teachings to invite blessings," commonly translated by others as the "secret" teachings (Penelope Quest in *Reiki for Life*: "The secret method of inviting happiness"[5]) is worth reflecting upon for a moment. Whilst the word "secret" is literally accurate, it should have a deeper resonance than the Western understanding of this word, which would generally refer to something classified or confidential, that you are not permitted to see or know: some closely guarded information, not for your eyes. What is being implied in the original Japanese context, however, as Stiene rightly notes, is something deeper, esoteric and spiritual in nature.[6] It is in fact the first call to mindfulness in the Precepts: to be aware, to explore the teachings deeply and rediscover your True Nature through the realisation and achievement of the state of enlightenment. The primary and most significant method to achieve this is through the practice of meditation.

Mikao Usui required that his students chant or repeat the Precepts every morning and evening. This process was designed to plant seeds of conscious awareness and reminds them to constantly bring to mind and attempt to live the Precepts in a meaningful way. They are, after all, a good road map for life. They are also a reminder to practice mindfulness meditation; *Be mindful about this in your heart/mind.* The requirement within the system to practice mindfulness, however, is not just something that should occur as a consequence of the chanting, after the fact. Awareness should also be applied – needs to be applied – to the chanting process itself. It is very easy, particularly for the Western mind, to slip into a chanting practice that becomes meaningless, hollow and lacking in focus as the mind is allowed to drift off. This needs to be avoided. Awareness (mind) is energy. Without mind, energy has nowhere to go and transformation can't take place.

One aspect of the Precepts that is not always given the importance that it deserves is the expression *Today only*, or as it is given in most other extant versions: *Just for today*. We should be clear that *today only, do not anger (or worry)* or *just for today, do not anger (or worry)* doesn't mean we should simply get on with our day-to-day activities as normal whilst putting off any anger and worry that we might have for another time. It means to pin consciousness into this very moment and be utterly aware of the moment. Anger and worry then find it extremely difficult to arise in an environment of focused awareness.

When we practice *anapanasati*, mindfulness of the breath, we are pinning our consciousness to the present moment; right *now*. When we develop our ability to stay in the present and become aware of the transient nature of our thoughts and our emotional states, we gain freedom from the attachments that are formed around the illusory nature of permanence of these transient phenomena. This freedom is profoundly liberating. As we focus on the breath, we discover that our emotions have a natural tendency to calm down, because we are not so focused on whatever would have led to their arising. We are less buffeted by life's swing of the pendulum from this experience to that experience, and we are more able to stay calm, centered and balanced. Thus, the arising of anger and worry, etc., becomes less likely to happen and with the development of awareness, insight naturally tends to arise; insight into our true nature of being and the true nature of reality. We start to be able to see everything and everyone as the passing phenomena that they really are, rather than fixed, solid and permanent, including ourselves. We start to appreciate the un-satisfactoriness and core-lessness of all that exists. Nothing is fixed. Nothing is permanent. Everything passes away. Impermanence in our day-to-day life is, however, masked by continuity. We see the continuous flow of the breath or the passing of the clouds in the sky and feel that this is a permanent state of being. We miss the fact that each breath is new. The old one is gone and finished with and useless. Continuity is the mask that impermanence hides behind, fooling us into believing in the fantasy of permanence. Likewise, the unsatisfactory nature of all phenomena is masked by change and movement. Before we have the chance to see how unsatisfactory something is, it is gone or transformed. We can also note that core-lessness, the inherent emptiness of all materialised forms, is hidden by compactness, and solidity. When we gain this awareness, we are much less likely to give way to destructive emotional states such as anger, etc., as we have a deeper and more profound engagement with the true nature of the manifest universe. We can start to see the emptiness of these emotions, how they are themselves simply passing mental events, and so we become less inclined to buy into them and allow them to control us and harm us.

Let us look at, *Today only, do not anger*: Anger is really an expression of ego and a lack of control. It is the product of a lack of insight, and ignorance of the true nature of reality. Life is not doing what we want it to do. *He shouldn't say that he should say this*, or *she shouldn't behave like that, she should behave like this* or *the government shouldn't be running the country that way, they should be running it this way.* Anger is always the product of us trying to impose upon the world how we think the world should be. If we're going to resolve our issues with anger, we need to let go of this need to control. We need to let go of this ego-driven idea that we know best; we know how the world and everyone and everything in it should be, that we can "concretise" it and fix it immutably in our own image. We do not know what is best for the world. We don't even know what is best for ourselves, let alone the rest of the world. Practicing mindfulness melts the need to control and allows us to accept the way things are right at this moment in time. It develops the mind of wisdom. It allows us to catch our mind before it goes on a rampage of self-destructive anger and frustration. Practicing Reiki, which develops our awareness of energy, gives us the ability to feel what harmful effects anger can create in the body in a way that perhaps non-Reiki practitioners cannot. When we do this, we can start to generate a field of compassion, for ourselves in the first instance, and then for the object of our intended anger or frustration. The development of our ability to release the need to control has profound implications for our Reiki healing work, as we shall see later.

Today only, do not worry: Worry arises out of our lack of ability to stay in the present moment. If we are in the moment, we appreciate and resonate on a deep level with the reality of the temporary nature of all phenomena. We see and notice that everything has a beginning and an end. Phenomena arises, has its moment and passes away. When we do not appreciate this, we form attachments to things, people, situations, etc., because we believe in the illusion of permanence. There is an internet meme that sums this up perfectly: *The bad news is: nothing lasts for ever. The good news is: nothing lasts for ever.* We need to develop the ability to hold everything with an open palm instead of a clenched fist. We spend so much of our time living in the past or the future, worry and restlessness become our constant companions. We look to the future and worry because we see it through the lens of our past: we impose upon it our past experiences and conditioning. Consequently, we become restless. As we learn to appreciate the reality of the transient nature of all things, we become less inclined to worry, as the object of our worry will also arise and pass away, and we find ourselves free of unnecessary suffering. Having an open palm allows everything to simply drift away. The clenched fist on the other hand will inevitably lead us on the road to worry, suffering and a life of pain.

Today only, be grateful: We need to appreciate the gift of life. When we practice Reiki and mindfulness, we start to release the energy of anger and other negative mind states and replace them with the energy of compassion (Reiki), insight and wisdom. As we increase our abilities to feel compassion for ourselves and appreciate our own lives, the more we start to respect and appreciate the lives of others. We start to feel our connectedness to all beings. When this happens, we can become one with universal consciousness as we realise on a deep level that everything is interconnected and implicit within everything is the entirety of the cosmos. If we were to take a simple glass of water, and ask ourselves *what is this?* We could simply reply that it is a glass of water. Where did that water come from? Maybe its source is in a river or a well. We can say then that implicit within the glass of water is the river or well. How did the water get into the river? It's possible that it fell as rain. We can say then that also within the glass of water, is the rain. Rain falls from clouds, so we can say that the clouds are in the glass of water. Of course, the clouds need the sky, so the sky is in the glass of water. We can go on. Eventually we realise that within that single glass of water is the whole cosmos. Within everything, is everything else. All is indeed one. This is true Reiki.

When Usui enjoins us to "practice diligently" he is asking us to put some effort into our practice of mindfulness and to commit to it: to be conscientious about our practice. We need to take some time out each day to develop our abilities to be mindful.

Be kind to yourself and others is obviously something that we should be doing, whether we practice Reiki or not. Sometimes, however, as we all know, this can be difficult. We can often be very hard on ourselves and unforgiving of our own shortcomings, let alone that of others. In the context of the practice of mindfulness, this Precept asks that we practice *metta bhavana. Metta* is the Pali word for "loving kindness" (all of the early Buddhist texts were recorded in the Pali language which is said to be the language of the historical Buddha[7]), and *bhavana* means cultivation or development. *Metta bhavana* therefore is the cultivation of loving kindness. In Japanese this is *Aijō no komotta kaihatsu,* but we will stay with the more widely known term of *metta bhavana*. All good mindfulness teachers will teach the cultivation of *metta*. *Metta* can be used to soften the breath during an *anapanasati* practice. We start the practice by sending loving energy inwards to ourselves, and then outwards to other beings. Research into the practice of *metta bhavana* has shown that regular practice has benefits ranging from a general sense of enhanced wellbeing to relief from illness and improved emotional and creative intelligence. As Dr Barbara Fredrickson of the University of North Carolina has said: "When people open their hearts to positive emotions, they seed their own growth in ways that transform them for the better."[8] We will return to the subject of the cultivation of *metta* later.

It should be clear that the Precepts are not simply something to chant each day but are a call to practice mindfulness meditation. Mindfulness is the foundations of the Reiki Precepts. Without practicing mindfulness meditation, you cannot expect to bring into manifestation these profound instructions for your life. In fact, without mindfulness, you are not really practicing Reiki at all. It is the warp and weft of the system. Let's now take a slight diversion into a meditation practice that develops our mindfulness in a classic Reiki-meditation context and brings in an aspect of practice called *samatha*.

According to German Reiki Master Frank Arjava Petter, there are Three Pillars in Reiki. These are *Gassho, Reiji-Ho* and Chiryo[9]: three simple techniques for connecting and working with the healing energy of Reiki. Unknown in the West until the publication of Petter's book *The Original Reiki Handbook of Dr Mikao Usui*, the Three Pillars are described as the foundation of the practice of Reiki. Let's look at the first of these Pillars: Gassho.[10]

When we put our hands together as if to pray, this is the *Gassho* mudra.[11] Most Reiki Masters acknowledge the importance of this *mudra*, and there is an expectation that most Reiki healing sessions would begin with the practitioner performing *Gassho*. This should last for about five minutes or so. The practice is said to help purify the energy of the surrounding space and help the practitioner enter into a state of mindful awareness.[12] In my own classes, my students are taught to do *Gassho* at the start of every healing session as a way to connect with the Reiki recipient and as an opportunity for them to center themselves and do a simple dedication for the benefit of the recipient. Of course, it's also a good practice, as Mikao Usui instructed, to sit in *Gassho* at the beginning and the end of the day when chanting the Reiki Precepts.[13] Sitting in *Gassho* is not just a traditional posture for chanting, centering yourself or purifying the energy of a space, however. It is also the basis of a powerful meditation practice in its own right.

When practicing *Gassho*, you should expect to sit for around 20 to 30 minutes. If you find it too difficult to sit for this length of time, especially if you are a beginner, then 10 minutes would be fine. You can always increase the amount of time later. Your hands come together at the heart and preferably at a height so that the exhaled breath will gently touch the fingertips. Your entire focus during the meditation should be on the point where both middle fingers meet.

The following meditation is a short introduction to the practice, but you can extend this as you wish, once you are familiar with it.

Gassho Meditation

Firstly, assume your meditation posture, close your eyes and place your hands in Gassho in front of your chest. Your arms and your hands should be relaxed. Release any tension that may creep in. Now run your mind over your body, checking your posture and releasing any tension that you find there with each out breath. Check your shoulders and release any tension that you find there also. Allow your spine to rest in its natural curve, but sit up straight, with your head balanced comfortably on your neck, as if there were a thread from the heavens holding it erect. If you are using a chair, make sure that you are not resting against the back of it and that your feet are planted firmly on the floor. If you have a physical problem and need the back support, then place a cushion or bolster there if necessary. Make sure that you are relaxed, alert and comfortable.

Go over your body one more time, from the crown of your head down to the tips of your toes, releasing any tension that you find, and allowing your body to sink down into gravity. Your posture will give you the sense of quiet dignity: poised and alert and perfectly stable.

Bring your attention to your breath. Follow your breath all the way in, and all the way out. Feel your belly rise and then fall with the breath. Sense your breath in other parts of your body. Really go into the experience of the breath. Where do you feel it? What does it feel like? Just observe it. You don't need to do anything with it. Just allow the breath to breathe itself, in and out.

If your mind wanders, this is okay. Just acknowledge this, let the thought go and bring your awareness back to the breath. Spend a few moments focusing on the breath and allowing the mind to settle.

When you are ready, you may open your eyes just a little. Keep them gently half open with a soft gaze and focus your attention on the tips of your fingers, where the two middle fingers meet. Keep your focus here and if thoughts come into your mind, again, simply acknowledge them and bring your focus back to your fingertips. Keep returning your focus to the tips of your middle fingers.

Don't try to achieve anything. Have no goal for this practice. Simply rest your awareness on your fingertips and try to become fully absorbed into this experience to the exclusion of everything else. You may find that the sensation of energy manifests at your fingers or on your palms or elsewhere in your body. Note this but keep your focus on your fingertips. Note whatever arises. But always return to your fingertips and allow your breath to be natural.

Be aware of any tendency for your head to tilt forwards. If this happens, again bring your head back into the upright position and allow your eyes to look down. There is no need to tilt the head.

Maintain your focus on your fingertips for a few more moments. Allow whatever arises to arise and then let it go.

Then slowly close your eyes and return your attention to your breath. Watch the breath going in and out. Feel the breath in your body. Feel the rise and fall of your belly. Keep your awareness on your breath for a few moments, noticing its effect on the rest of the body.

Now bring your awareness back into the room that you are in. Become aware of the weight of your body connected to the earth. Take a few deep breaths and in your own time, gently open your eyes and lower your hands.

There are two components to this meditation that are worth drawing attention to. The first of these is the mindfulness aspect where we are being asked to observe reality: the rise and fall of the breath and the awareness of sensations at our fingertips (and elsewhere in the body as they arise), as well as an awareness of the fingertips themselves. This is classic insight meditation: awareness of things as they are. The second aspect of the meditation is called *samatha*. *Samatha* means "tranquillity." A *samatha* meditation requires us to become single-pointed in our observation of the object of the meditation (the fingertips in this instance). The state of tranquillity or bliss that can arise due to a *samatha* practice occurs when we are utterly absorbed or concentrated into the object of the meditation to the exclusion of all else. Essentially our mind becomes tranquilized: it becomes soft, pliable, malleable and expansive. However, the benefits of a *samatha* practice are not easily transferable to our every day, moment to moment lives. You can't stay in a permanent state of bliss due to a *samatha* practice. Life will always pull you out of it. *Samatha* meditations are incapable of leading you to a realisation of the state of enlightenment on their own. *Samatha* is a skill that is necessary in the practice of *vipassana*, however, and *vipassana* can most certainly lead you to a realisation of the state of enlightenment. *Vipassana*, as we noted in the previous chapter, is another name for mindfulness meditation.

Although it is possible to practice *samatha* and *vipassana* separately, the Buddha gave no such recommendation, and to do so would not be in alignment with the Buddha's way of thinking. It is better to practice both simultaneously. In this way we can deepen our ability to become absorbed to a very high degree in the meditation subject, and at the same time develop our faculty of insight by accepting and noting the way things are right now. *Samatha* and *vipassana* are separated only by their end-goal: the purpose of *samatha* is to calm the mind. The purpose of *vipassana* is to gain insight. *Vipassana* will of course also lead to a calming of the mind, but that is not its function. Essentially, the fixed unchanging qualities of our *samatha* meditation object reveal themselves to be impermanent and unsatisfactory when viewed through a *vipassana* lens, thus enabling us to let it go, breaking our attachments to the world of form and materiality.

As a form of *samatha/vipassana* meditation the objectives of the *Gassho* practice are to still the mind and bring it into a state of one-pointed concentration on the fingertips and the accompanying sensations due to the Reiki flow. This will bring about a state of profound tranquillity and bliss. As we continue in our absorbed state on the experience of our fingertips, we acknowledge whatever arises during the practice. We note the way the sensations of energy change, move and fluctuate. There is a sense of impermanence about these sensations. They are not fixed. They are in flux. We acknowledge and accept our mind's wandering and then bring it back to the focus. We recognize, too, that our mind, our thought process is also in a state of flux. We might notice a bird singing, a car passing by, the feel of the breeze against our face. All of these are inclusive within the meditation experience. We note them and let them go, in the same way that we note the ever-changing nature of the experience of energy at our fingertips. There is nothing to hold on to. Everything arises and passes away. As our *samatha* experience deepens over time, we start to "screen out" external distractions, but still, we are deeply aware of the impermanence of our meditation object: our fingertips and the accompanying sensations. Our fingertips are an aspect of our physical body. By reflecting deeply on the fingertips, we are naturally led into a reflection on our whole body and its state of impermanence.

Chanting the Precepts

It is worth looking at the practice of chanting the Precepts from a mindfulness perspective. As I have said, chanting the Precepts helps to plant a seed in the consciousness to prompt us to be aware and mindful during our normal daily activities that we need to bring to life the true essence of the Precepts. However, the Precepts are said to work on another level also. It is claimed that in Japanese they contain something called *kotodama,* which is a Shinto word expressing the idea that words have spiritual power in their own right. By chanting them, it is believed that we are directing our minds in a specific energetic direction. Frank Petter noted in *This Is Reiki*:

> *The power of a kotodama lies in the pronunciation, the sound/ frequency, and therefore, it must be spoken to reveal its power.... [The Reiki Precepts] are to be recited in their original language, in Japanese, to release their power.* (Petter, 2012)[14]

It is claimed that if the Precepts are recited correctly therefore, even if there is no understanding of the words it can have a profound effect on the mind and body, removing impurities and creating a store house of positive energy. It is also claimed that the same vibrational effect is not created when the Precepts are recited in translated form. However, some have claimed that they have found great benefit when chanting them in another language such as English. Wadie, one of my Egyptian students, noted this: "I chant them once a day (sometimes in the morning, evening or at night) because they make a difference. It's like my mind is being conditioned by them. I chant them in English because they make sense to me in this language. I learned them in English and that's what I choose to stick with." Whether or not the Precepts do indeed contain *kotodama* is open to debate. Some find benefit in chanting them in their original Japanese, others find benefit in chanting them in their own language, some (such as myself) find no benefit from chanting them in any language beyond their usefulness as aids to a mindfulness practice.

There is also some controversy amongst linguists over the concept of *kotodama* in Japanese, and it has been stated that the resurgence of *kotodama* in Japanese culture is a throwback to the 1930s and the nationalism that existed at that time based on the idea of the primacy of Japanese amongst the world's languages.[15] However, regardless of the language in which the

Precepts are chanted, it is worth emphasising the need to be mindful of the precise words as you chant them.

If you wish to have a go at chanting the Precepts, firstly assume your meditation posture and focus your attention on your *hara*. Still your mind as much as you can. Spend a moment or two focusing on your breath. If you have it, you can visualise the second Reiki symbol at your Third Eye for a few moments (if you haven't got the Reiki symbols yet, get in touch with your Reiki Master and take the second level! You won't regret it). This symbol has a powerful effect on helping to still the mind. Don't worry if you don't have it, the practice is still highly beneficial without it. Whether you use the symbol or not, try to be present in the moment.

Draw the breath in smoothly through the nose and then intone the Precepts in a low deep voice whilst breathing out through the mouth. Vocalise the words slowly and strongly, with your full attention on them. Be mindful of the sound; the effect of the sound at your vocal cords and in your *hara* and anywhere else in your body. Try to let each sound fill and vibrate throughout your whole body. Make sure you pronounce each word clearly, ensuring you don't slur them together. Be mindful of every moment and every sound that you utter and the effect that these sounds have on you and your surroundings.

Chapter 3

Meditation with the Reiki Symbols & Mantras

Much is said about the healing functions of the Reiki symbols (*shirushi* in Japanese). You can find them discussed in this context in almost every book and website ever written about Reiki and dozens of techniques are given for their use. Rarely, however, are they discussed in relation to their use as meditation objects, which is unfortunate as this is their primary function. When it is discussed, it is often in the context of simply helping someone connect to specific qualities or frequencies of energy.[1] This is peripheral and useful once again, only in a hands-on healing context (though even in this context, it is debatable that "connecting to different frequencies of energy" is what is happening[2]). When I teach about the symbols in a class, I am at great pains to emphasize that they are not just for use in healing. As their origins are within esoteric Buddhism, they are, like their Buddhist counterparts, used principally as devices for bringing stillness and focus to the mind, to help the meditator access different aspects of their own being and to help guide them on their journey towards enlightenment. In working with the symbols as meditation devices, the practitioner returns to the essence of their True Nature or Buddha Nature from which they had been unconsciously alienated. The practice helps to re-center daily life as we move into a space of reintegration with the Absolute.

Symbols can be regarded as a midway point between the external physical world and what is deeply embedded within. They are one of the ways in which we can approach our True Nature, by internalising our consciousness and allowing the inherent qualities and functions of the symbols to lead us to higher states of awareness. By using symbols, we can raise our consciousness and thus potentially achieve or realise the state of enlightenment.

This approach to the symbols was emphasized by Frans Stiene in his book *Reiki Insights* when he said:

> *The symbols are tools to help us to rediscover our own hidden inner light, our Reiki, our true self.... By meditating on the symbols again and again and again, we start to slowly peel away our layers of ignorance, our anger and worry; this in turn will lay bare our hidden inner great bright light.... This is also why the symbols and mantras were tools for meditation, meant to help us go within. However, over time they have become very externalised and now often are used only during hands-on healing sessions.* (Stiene, 2017)[3]

As meditative tools it is worth spending some time trying to understand the symbols and the *mantras* (often translated as *jumon* in Japanese, though this can have the connotation of being associated with folk-magic spells) that are traditionally associated with them. We must, however, be aware that in the West we have a need for things to make sense and have a consciously intellectual underpinning approach to the symbols, around which we can anchor our practice. This need can often block our understanding, as esoteric symbols resonate deeply at the level of the unconscious and their inner or secret aspects are often beyond the realms of logic and rationality and the parameters of the conscious mind. The symbols act as a bridge between two levels of truth: the relative and the absolute. We can say that relative truth is the way that the world appears to exist, and absolute truth is the way the world actually exists. That said and from our place within the world of relative truth, we should still endeavor to piece together what we can about the symbols to give us a starting point in our practice with them.

A cautionary note, however, first: Whilst the system of Reiki is very much a Japanese creation, the energy that we also call Reiki is not. This energy is universal (it's there in its name; Reiki means "universal life force energy"). It's not limited by culture. This energy is the common birth right of everyone and everything in existence, regardless of how we view or understand the nature of life and our part in it, and regardless of how we understand the subtle energy system of the human body. Reiki energy is as much a part of the subtle anatomy of an Indian yogi who views this energy in terms of a system of *marma* points, *nadi* channels and *chakras*, as it is a Japanese Aikido practitioner who understands energy in terms of the three *tandens* and their associated elixir fields. In keeping with the practices of many writers on the subject of other oriental practices (*Qi Gong*, or *Ki Ko* in Japanese, for instance), I will at times be referring to the relationship between the Reiki symbols and the *chakra* system, firstly, because it is eminently relevant, and secondly because it's just easier. This isn't to imply that the system of Reiki is anything other than a Japanese system, though the cultural and spiritual tools and methods that Mikao Usui drew upon in his formulation of the system are open to extensive debate.[4]

So, let's start by taking these symbols apart to get a better understanding of what they are all about.

The *mantras* associated with the symbols are frequently misapplied and referred to as the names of the symbols (Symbol 1: *Choku Rei*, Symbol 2: *Sei Hei Ki* Symbol 3: *Hon Sha Ze Sho Nen*, Symbol 4: *Dai Ko Myo*). They are, however, entirely separate devices for invoking the same energetic qualities as the visual symbols[5] (which I will be referring to by their numbers). In a healing context, if we wish to focus the energy, for instance, we can either draw Symbol 1 or repeat its associated *mantra*. Both devices do the same thing. Better still would be to draw the symbol and repeat the *mantra* simultaneously as both devices support and enhance the effects and attributes of the other.

The word *mantra* can be broken down into two parts: *man* which means mind, and *tra* which means vehicle. A *mantra* therefore is a vehicle for the mind. It is a sound that can help you enter a deep state of meditation. Just as you plant a seed, you plant *mantras* in the fertile soil of your mind, which in time can grow and enable you to expand your consciousness into new ways of being. The *mantras* associated with the Reiki symbols can plant energetic imprints that allow you to access certain qualities on a much deeper level.

These mantric devices are the auditory equivalent of the visual symbols, and it goes without saying that just like the Reiki Precepts are said to contain *kotodama* (spiritual power), so do the Reiki symbols. To be able to engage fully with the symbols as objects of meditation we should try to understand the symbols and associated *mantras* a little more deeply than the tip-of-the-iceberg definitions they are commonly known for in hands-on-healing. According to Frank Petter: "These Symbols came from India to Tibet where they were copied by Chinese monks. From China they made their way to Japan" (Petter, 1997).[6] There is clearly an indication here of an origin for, or recognition of the symbols within esoteric Buddhism and there can be little doubt that Usui, in creating what came to be known as Reiki was influenced quite substantially by this over his inclusion of symbols into his system. The use of *mantra* alongside the practice of meditating on symbols or *yantras* (visual meditation devices) is very common in many schools of esoteric Buddhism.

It has been claimed by Reiki Master Chris Marsh that Usui introduced the symbols to the system some 13 years after he introduced the mantric forms (approximately in 1910 and 1923 respectively)[7]. However, as James Deacon quite rightly points out in quoting Reiki Master Jiro Kozuki it may well have been not so much a case of Usui introducing or "creating" the symbols, or importing them from outside of his system, but more likely that he selected symbols that were already present within the system.[8] Their simplified meanings that we are all familiar with (Symbol 1 for increasing energy, Symbol 2 for mental and emotional healing, Symbol 3 for distant healing and Symbol 4 for initiating others into the system) may have been Usui's attempt to make these complex meditation devices accessible to those that needed them for their work in using the system as a simple hands-on therapy. Reiki Master Hiroshi Doi has claimed that the symbols were to be used as no more than "training wheels" and then dispensed with after the practitioner had internalised their primary healing functions: "Try to move away from the symbols when you have developed the ability to use them properly" (Doi, 2000).[9] It is actually more likely the case that when a practitioner has internalised the basic functions of the symbols, that their real journey of exploration with them has just begun (though it has to be said, the symbols are only tools and we should avoid any undue attachment to them).

It's worth noting that spiritual symbols are not "invented" or "made up." You can't just sit down and doodle your own on a notepad over coffee. Spiritual symbols are discovered within the infinite void of the Absolute or the Universal Energy Field by the highly realised minds of very advanced spiritual practitioners. They look the way they do because of the laws of something called "form" or "space" energy. This means on a basic level that if you want to generate the energy of "circle" you can't do that by drawing a square. You must always draw a circle. The Reiki symbols, therefore, were not created by Mikao Usui, he discovered them, either through his own meditative practices or from some other source. The symbols simply express qualities and attributes that are already fundamentally part of our own True Nature, so in discovering the symbols, Usui was simply externalising and bringing into conscious manifestation, tools for all of us to use as an aid in realising our True Nature once more.

Associations have been made between the Reiki symbols and various Buddhist deities and *Bodhisattvas*[10] (*Bosatsu* in Japanese) by Reiki Master Dave King,[11] and others. Most specifically with Amida (Amitabha) Buddha; the Buddha of Infinite Light.[12] It is said that Amida "shed a tear of compassion upon recognizing the suffering of all sentient beings, and from this tear was born a special emanation of the Bodhisattva Kannon (Avalokiteshvara in Sanskrit)..."[13] (Pearson, 2018). Avalokiteshvara is the *Bodhisattva* of Compassion and from a Christian perspective has often been equated with the Virgin Mary. In the practice of Reiki, we do not work with Buddhist deities or *Bodhisattvas*, however, there are tantric meditations of the Vajrayana and Mahayana schools of Buddhism that involve the self-generation of Avalokiteshvara. In a self-generation practice the practitioner essentially "becomes" the deity or *Bodhisattva* that is the focus of his/her practice and embodies all of their innate qualities. It's very possible that Mikao Usui, given his adherence to esoteric Buddhism (most likely Pure Land Buddhism, as he is buried in a Pure Land cemetery [others have suggested that he was Tendai or Shingon, though this is all highly speculative][14]), may well have been involved in such practices prior to or during his formulation of his spiritual system. For those who wish to pursue working with Amida Buddha in his various forms and explore the concept of self-generation to enhance their understanding and journey with Reiki, check out *A Practice of Consciousness Transference Involving Amitabha (The Gateway to Sukhavati)* written by the Fifth Dalai Lama, and *The Practice Called Opening the Eyes* translated by Lama Zopa Rinpoche.[15]

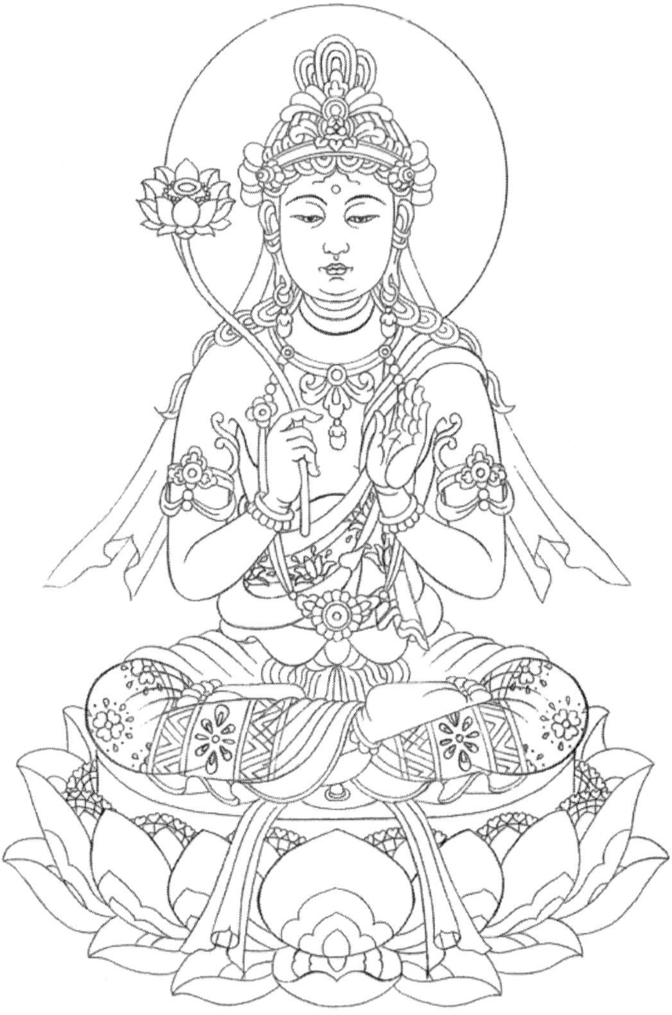

Associations with Buddhist deities are likely to have a direct correlation with the visual framework of the various symbols. The way the symbols are perceived as meditation or healing devices is of great significance, as it is in this that we find their real depth and meaning. It is important to keep in mind that as Reiki is a secular method, the references here to Buddhist deities and *Bodhisattvas* are provided simply to anchor awareness of key attributes and universal qualities during your meditation on the Reiki symbols.

It is also worth emphasising that the *mantras* are equally important in the practice of Reiki. If we think of the symbols as *yantras* or as a manifestation of a *yantra,* we can see that *mantra* is essential to their use. *Mantras* and *yantras* are interchangeable in many ways; both fulfilling pretty much the same functions. However, whereas a *mantra* can be used on its own, a *yantra* requires the use of a *mantra* alongside it. If you think for a moment in terms of the use of *yantra* (or symbol) to embody the quality of a particular deity (which is the usual practice within Hinduism), we can see that the *mantra* is the deity him or herself whilst the *yantra* is the body of the deity. So, in a sense, when we use *mantra* with the symbols, we are in fact "installing" the quality that we want within the structure of the symbol (*yantra*),[16] but at the same time it is a quality that is inherent within it; that it has a natural predisposition towards. The *mantra* is not activating the symbol, as some in the West believe.

> *Inseparable from yantras are the subtle vibrations which help to intensify their power.... The inner dynamics of the yantra can never be understood in isolation from the system of sound dynamics, as the two combine to make up the complete 'definition'.... The yantra-mantra complex is basically an equation that unites space (akasa), which in its gross form appears as shapes, and vibrations, which in their finite forms occur as the spoken or written word.* (Khana, 2003)[17]

Symbol 1: The Power or Focus Symbol

Let's work on the highly probable assumption as James Deacon has pointed out in reference to Reiki Master Jiro Kozuki that Usui took something that was already within the system and developed it for use as a healing tool. In this scenario there are two possibilities: that Usui simply took the symbol as is and simplified its meaning (or focused on one aspect of its meaning) for use in a healing context, or more likely the symbol was extracted from some larger meditative device or *yantra*, i.e., Symbol 1 being a visual component within a larger *yantra*.[18]

If we look at the meaning of the *mantra Choku Rei* we find different possible meanings. These meanings depend on the *kanji*, or Japanese characters, used to write the *mantra Choku Rei*. It can mean *imperial command or edict* or *direct spirit* or *supreme spiritual emptiness* (the Absolute).[19] All of these meanings are deeply interrelated. Certainly, we can see that in a healing context, the idea of an *imperial command* is useful, perhaps signifying a divine command to *put the power here* or *focus the power here*. It has an external quality about it and certainly the experience of most when using this device in a healing context is that it does indeed *put the power here*. It is worth noting, however, that Symbol 1 and *Choku Rei* are related to Seishi *Bosatsu* (*Bodhisattva*).[20] On a spiritual level, when focusing on and doing practices associated with Seishi (such as a self-generation practice), we do so to develop power, or the capacity to be effective, confident, assertive. i.e., *put the power here*; to assert our truth. It is a command from Seishi whom we are in a sense embodying when we use Symbol 1 and its *mantra*. Seishi often appears in Buddhist iconography as one of the main attendants of Amida Buddha and represents the power of wisdom. The other attendant to Amida is Kannon, or Avalokiteshvara embodying, as we have seen, the quality of compassion.

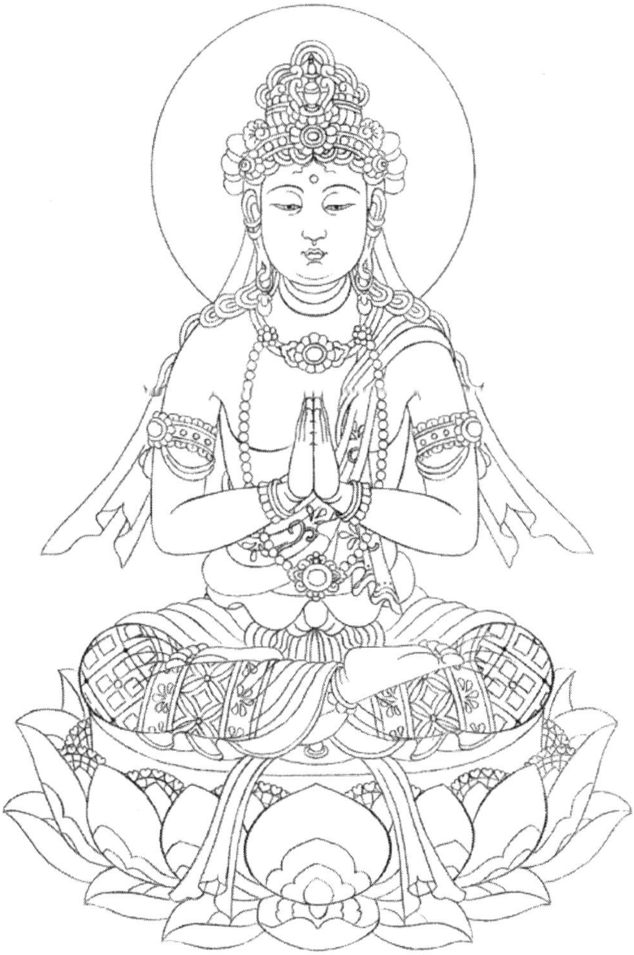

If we wish to explore Symbol 1 and its *mantra* further, we must now turn to other understandings and the concept of *direct spirit*. So, what do we mean by *direct spirit*? According to the research of James Deacon in quoting Masahisa Goi,[21] founder of the religious group Byakko Shinkokai, *direct spirit* refers to the power of God, the supreme being. Goi writes in *The Future of Mankind*:

> *chokurei, [is] the image of God working in this world of mankind....*[22]

We ask then "what is God?" Perhaps the omniscient state of oneness? As Jalal ad-Din Muhammad Rumi, the Sufi mystic and poet said "I searched for God and found only myself. I searched for myself and found only God." The divine, the state of oneness, is our own True Nature: our Buddha Nature. However, as Goi states, *Choku Rei* is the *image* of God, not God him/herself. It is something that points to the divine, to our Buddha Nature. It is an aid to help us find or realise enlightenment (the Absolute).

Let's return to Rumi's search for God once more: "I looked into my own heart and there I saw Him; He was nowhere else." If we wind Symbol 1 through the body's subtle energy system, we find that the termination of the final turn of the spiral ends in the center of the chest at the Heart chakra or the elixir field for the middle *tanden*. This is no coincidence.

If we view Symbol 1 as a *yantra*, or as the central component within a larger *yantra* we must acknowledge that, as with all *yantras*, at the center is something called a *bindu*: a point or dot symbolising the cosmos prior to its creation. The *bindu* stands between manifestation and the unmanifest, between actuality and potentiality. Sometimes within a *yantra*, this is physically drawn as a dot and sometimes it is simply implied. In the case of Symbol 1, the *bindu* point exists at the termination of the spiral at the Heart chakra. It is the point to which our consciousness should lead and ultimately merge with it.

The function of a *yantra* is to internalise consciousness and transcend the ordinary mind. *Yantra* meditations can work from the outer limits inwards to the center (symbolic of the deepening concentration and absorption of the meditator), or from the center outwards (symbolic of the expansion of the cosmos from its origination point). We could say that in meditating on Symbol 1, as we move from the outer edges to the central *bindu*, we are moving towards the single point of samadhi and in moving from the center outwards we are moving from the ego-centered state to the enlightened state. It is more usual, however, to move from the outer edges of the symbol to the center: bringing the mind to a single point of absorption within the symbol.

Although Symbol 1 can be used as a healing device, its primary function is as a meditation device. In terms of healing therefore, when we use the symbol to *put the power here,* it is not referring to the power of some external entity or being, or from "up there" in the Universal Energy Field. It is the power of our own True Nature (as embodied in Seishi *Bosatsu*). It is the state of enlightenment manifesting: oneness manifesting within the state of duality. In a sense the symbol is acting as an intermediary between relative and ultimate truth. It also acts like a magnifying glass: amplifying and focusing energy into a laser-like beam.

As the symbol relates to the concept of Buddhahood, it can be seen then that the *mantra Choku Rei* and the visual Symbol 1 are both tools for transcending duality and realising our innate quality of enlightenment. It is not simply for helping us to realise our "true nature" as a dualistically orientated person, but to help us transcend the very concept of duality and realise our True Nature as one with the universe: the macrocosm within the microcosm or our inherent Buddha Nature. Ultimately, this is in fact the goal of the whole Reiki system and was stated by Mrs Takata in her very first Reiki class in Hilo, Hawaii, in 1938 when she said the system of Reiki expressed the concept: "the universe is as I am; I am as the universe is" and related this to the expression "direct spirit" (Choku Rei).[23] Symbol 1 then encapsulates and synthesises the concept of the achievement of Buddhahood in a very powerful way.

As Shunryū Suzuki has said:

> *to be a human being is to be a Buddha. Buddha nature is just another name for human nature, our true human nature. Thus, even though you do not do anything, you are actually doing something. You are expressing yourself. You are expressing your true nature. Your eyes will express; your voice will express; your demeanour*

> *will express. The most important thing is to express your true nature in the simplest, most adequate way and to appreciate it in the smallest existence.* (Suzuki, 1970)[24]

This is the goal to which meditating on Symbol 1 and its associated *mantra* should lead.

Symbol 2: The Mental/Emotional or Harmony Symbol

The *mantra Sei Hei Ki* can be translated as follows:

Sei relates to birth or essential quality, becoming or coming to be, the true nature of the mind.

Hei signifies equilibrium balance, tranquillity, peaceful.

Heiki refers to a calm and tranquil undisturbed mind.

Ki is energy, spiritual energy, life energy or air/wind/atmosphere.

So, the function of the symbol/*mantra* complex is to enable us to discover our mind's original nature or essential quality. It is a state of balance, calm and blissful tranquillity. In a healing context we could say that it is the energy that brings tranquillity which is the essential nature of the mind.

In recent years it has become widely accepted that Symbol 2 is likely derived from the seed syllable *hrih* (*kiriku* in Japanese)[25] as expressed in the Siddham script (Siddham originally came from southern India, eventually spreading through China and then into Japan). A seed syllable is a glyph, derived from a *mantra*, that is thought to contain spiritual connections to the origination of things. The *hrih* is the core seed syllable for Amida Buddha (and thus for Kannon/Avalokiteshvara, as an emanation of Amida), therefore suggesting a relationship for Symbol 2 to the boundless and unceasing qualities of Amida's wisdom mind, heart of compassion and infinite bliss. *Hrih* is also the seed syllable for the Lotus Family of Buddhas[26] of which Amida is the head and to which human beings belong. The Lotus Family is linked to the transmutation of desire or attachment (which is the process of mental and emotional healing that we attempt to instigate with our use of Symbol 2 in a healing context). Symbol 2 and *hrih* have a strong visual resemblance. However, we must be mindful of the script that we are referencing when making visual comparisons. Although there clearly is something of a visual correspondence between *hrih* (see figure 8) when written in Siddham, there is much more of a visual correspondence with *hrih* in the Tibetan Uchen script (see figure 9). In fact, Symbol 2 has a strong visual resemblance to the individual elements of the entire *mantra Om Ah Hum Hrih*[27] in Uchen, which is used extensively in dedications to, and tantric self-generation practices of Avalokiteshvara/Amida Buddha. On close examination it is clear that Symbol 2 has a much closer visual relationship to elements of *om ah hum* than it does to *hrih*. It is very possible therefore that Symbol 2 is related not just to *hrih* but to the complete *mantra* that is used by adherents to fully embody the qualities associated with Avalokiteshvara/Amida. Like Symbol 1, Symbol 2 may have been extracted from a larger meditative device or *yantra*, rather than existing as a simple stand-alone symbol.

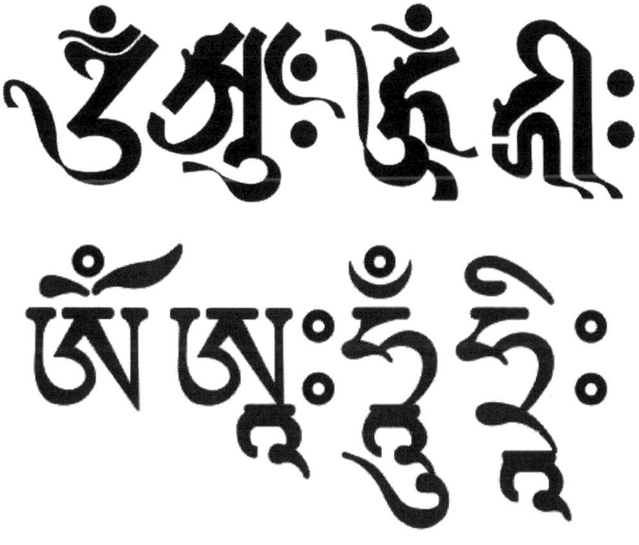

We know Symbol 2 within a healing context as the "mental/emotional symbol" and it is with this in mind that we can see that there is a relationship between the seed syllables *Om, Ah* and *Hum* as they relate to the Third Eye, Throat and Heart chakras (with Symbol 1 sitting at the Crown). The *mantra Sei Hei Ki* (and thus Symbol 2) conveys the essence of these seed syllables. When the symbol (or originating *yantra*) is meditated on, the mind and consciousness can reach a deep state of relaxation and one-pointed absorption or concentration. As the mind becomes more focused and rests at peace, the body, speech and mind are also purified. This is the process of mental and emotional healing.

As we have seen, the seed syllable *hrih,* has a relationship with the Lotus Family of Buddhas, with Amida at its head. With this in mind, we can also see that the *mantra Om Ah Hum* represents the Three *Kayas* of the Lotus Family.[28] The Three *Kayas* are the foundation and realisation of the whole of the esoteric Buddhist path and express different manifestations of the enlightened mind; mapping out a route that an aspirant or devotee can take to a realisation of their True Nature. The Three *Kayas* are: the *Dharmakaya* which relates to Dainichi Buddha[29]; the Supreme or Sun Buddha (*Om*), the *Sambhogakaya* which relates to Kannon/Avalokiteshvara (*Ah*) and the *Nirmanakaya* which relates to any great spiritual teacher such as Shakyamuni Buddha, Padmasambhava or Kukai (*Hum*). It could be said that *Sei Hei Ki* is the vehicle and the map for our spiritual journey through these three qualities or states of being and non-being of the fully enlightened mind, known as the Three *Kayas*.

The *Dharmakaya* is our ultimate destination on the spiritual path, which as we have seen is signified by the *bindu* point of Symbol 1 at the Heart chakra – the balance point in the human subtle energy system. It's worth reflecting on the fact that the name of the Heart chakra is *Anahata* and that this is also another name for *Om*; the "unstruck sound"; the sound of creation.[30] *Om* was the first impulse to emerge from the silence of the Absolute, or the field of Pure Potentiality. It is the formless form; has no substance and is devoid of all concepts, including existence and non-existence. It has a direct equivalence with Dainichi Buddha (the *Dharmakaya*) and embodies our true state of being.

Ah is the *Sambhogakaya* and relates to Avalokiteshvara, another manifestation of Amida Buddha. The *Sambhogakaya* is the bridge between the formless and the world of form. Like the *Dharmakaya* it is implicit and ever present in all beings; we simply need to bring it into realisation. The *Sambhogakaya*, as the syllable *Ah* clearly indicates, sitting as it does at the throat, has to do with how we communicate or express ourselves, not just verbally but in all forms. When we express compassion (not ordinary human compassion but the infinite unconditioned compassion of the Absolute), this is an aspect of *Sambhogakaya*. So, the *Sambhogakaya* is the realisation or manifestation of a blissful, beginning-less and endless transcendental feeling or quality of compassion for all beings. It has a non-dualistic quality to it: it is not "me" feeling compassion for "you." There is no me. There is no you. There is just compassion.

Hum is the *Nirmanakaya*. This is the physical flesh-and-blood being that has manifested in the world to show all beings the way to enlightenment and freedom from suffering. Just like everyone else, however, they are subject to old-age, sickness and death. The historical Buddha is an example of the *Nirmanakaya*. It's believed that at death, a *Nirmanakaya* Buddha can take on the form of a *Sambhogakaya* Buddha.

Our journey with Symbol 2 in its simple form as a healing mechanism, but more importantly as a more complex meditative device, is to purify the body, speech and mind and so lose our attachments to negative tendencies, obsessions and excessive desires, thus leading to an embodiment of the qualities of the *Nirmanakaya*, and eventually to a realisation of the state of infinite bliss as we merge into the field of the Absolute as expressed through the form of Amida or Dainichi Buddha (the termination point of Symbol 1).

Symbol 3: The Distant or Connection Symbol

The third symbol in the system of Reiki is not a symbol at all. It is Japanese writing in the form of *kanji*. *Kanji* is one of the three systems of Japanese writing and is based on a system of symbols that represent different words or concepts, so that they can have different meanings depending on their context.[31] With Symbol 3 therefore we have a much greater chance of a deeper understanding of the meanings associated with it. We can after all, simply read it. It is less a symbol in the classic sense of the word, and more the written form of a *mantra*.

It has been claimed that Usui "invented" or "designed" this symbol.[32] It has also been suggested that the symbol is possibly based on the development of Taoist charms and talismans[33] because it looks a bit like them or is based on the design of Buddhist *stupas*[34] (a *stupa* is "a Buddhist commemorative monument usually housing sacred relics associated with the Buddha or other saintly persons."[35]) because it looks a bit like them, but this is all just grasping at straws. If it were a symbol in the classic sense, then such origins might be vaguely credible. But really, even though in a healing context it is used as if it were a symbol, it really isn't. It's a sentence: a written *mantra*.

A number of people have analyzed the *kanji* structure of this symbol/*mantra* to ascertain its deeper meaning and then boiled these meanings down into a simple sentence. James Deacon has said that the symbol can be translated as essentially meaning: "Correct Thought (/Correct Mindfulness) is the essence of being."[36] Frans Stiene has given his version as: "My original self/ true self is a correct thought."[37] These versions are very close to each other; and say pretty much the same thing. They are on the whole good definitions (though I would argue that thought or the process of thinking has very little to do with the concept of True Self or Essence of Being). The problem, however, is that both versions boil down a highly complex philosophical construction into a pat, throw-away definition. If you want to truly discover where this symbol may lead, it is important to keep in mind the various complex multi-faceted characteristics of it as much as possible, and not reduce it to a simple definition that really leads nowhere.

Firstly, let's look at the meaning of the individual *kanji*:

Hon means source or origin or true source.

Sha means person, the one.

Ze means right or true or correct.

Sho means correct or exact, true or straight.

Nen means thought, idea, wish, feeling.

But we can go deeper than this and start to take apart some of the syllables themselves. If we look at just the bottom part of *Hon* for instance, we get another aspect of the *kanji*. The bottom part of the *Hon* means "ancient," "wise" or "wisdom."[38]

James Deacon on his *Reiki Pages* started to go beyond these simple definitions for Symbol 3 when he noted in relation to some forms of Japanese Reiki: "Symbol 3 is seen as representing the transcendent 'oneness' within the practitioner, and the realisation that there is no separation between the two people sharing the phenomenon of giving-receiving Reiki."[39] So we could say that its primary function (the realisation of our transcendent oneness with all that is) is pointing to its secondary function (distant healing). However, in some respects, we need to drop the secondary function (distant healing) altogether if we are to get to grips with this complex device.

> *In looking at the translation of this mantra we can already see that it has nothing to do with distance healing. In fact, the opposite is true; it is about rediscovering that there is no distance at all! It points straight to discovering our True Self.* (Stiene, 2014)[40]

This symbol has a much more sophisticated and complex story to tell. Bronwen and Frans Stiene have pointed out that this symbol/*mantra* is often linked to the *Bodhisattva* Kannon/ Avalokiteshvara.[41] More than this, however, it is a signifier for the Three *Kayas* and thus has a profound relationship with Symbol 2.

We have already seen how *Om Ah Hum* is the essence of form – our true essence (body, speech and mind). This is the *Hon* of Symbol 3. So, we can see that embedded within Symbol 3, is Symbol 2 (to put it simply). *Sha* means person. Who is this person? It is you, me, "I." It is pointing to our own inner wisdom. *Ze* means right or true or correct. Another word for *Ze* from the Buddhist canon is *vajra*.[42] The *vajra* represents Amida Buddha (Limitless Light). It also represents the purity and indestructability of the Buddha's teachings, and relates back to Symbol 1 which expresses the concept of indestructible truth and power as embodied in the form of Seishi *Bosatsu*, who is often depicted wielding a *vajra*. Amida Buddha or Seishi is the one who can help us or guide us to our own True Nature. *Sho* also means true or correct but in this instance the *kanji* relates to the truth of our own heart of compassion. *Nen* means thought, idea, wish. So *Nen* relates to a true wish or blessing coming from the heart (*Sho*).[43] In a sense then we can say that Symbol 3 is a narrative or description of our spiritual journey via the vehicle of Symbol 2 that leads to a realisation of Symbol 1 (and eventually Symbol 4).

When we work with Symbol 3, we need to keep in mind all these definitions as we contemplate it.

Symbol 4: The Master Symbol[44]

Symbol 4; the Master symbol, exists widely outside of the context of Reiki. It is very well known in martial arts circles and can be found in Buddhist temples in Japan; one of them being the temple at the foot of Mt Kurama; the mountain on which Usui had a moment of *satori* (an enlightenment experience) that fundamentally reshaped his spiritual practice.[45] Again, although Symbol 4 is used as if it were a symbol, like Symbol 3, it actually isn't. It's a sentence; the Japanese form of a *mantra*.

Let's look at what the separate *kanji* of this symbol mean:

Dai means big or great.

Ko means ray, light, shine or radiance.

Myo means clarity, brightness, clearness, light or *mantra*.

Komyo means hope, bright future, glory.

So, we could say that *Dai Ko Myo* essentially means "The great light of clarity (enlightenment)." It is said to be embodied in the image of the Buddha holding a bowl of fire above his head. Another interpretation of *Dai Ko Myo* is "The *mantra* of the great light."

It has been claimed that Symbol 4 is associated with Dainichi Buddha (also known as Maha Vairocana).[46] In this sense therefore, as Dainichi is the supreme expression of our final state of transcendence; the realisation of our innate Buddha nature, *Dai Ko Myo* has a direct relationship with Symbol 1. As we move towards the implied *bindu* at the center of the symbol, we discover or become one with our *Dai Ko Myo*. In a sense therefore, as we start our journey with the symbols in Reiki, we find that Symbol 1 is pointing to Symbol 4, which is our final destination: *Choku Rei* to *Dai Ko Myo*. We can also see that *Dai Ko Myo* has a relationship with the *Dharmakaya* as embodied within Dainichi Buddha as was discussed in relation to Symbol 2.

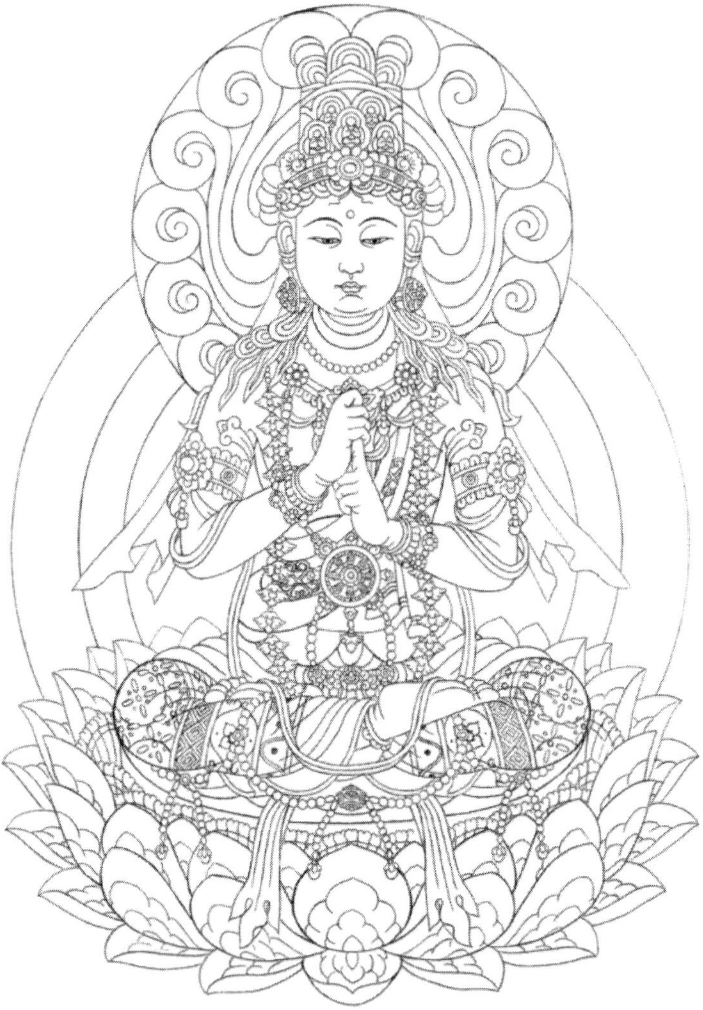

Let's get back to the *kanji* and look at them in terms of their Sanskrit equivalents:

Dai (Jp) is *Maha* (Sk).

Ko (Jp) is *Prabha* (Sk).

Myo (Jp) is *Surya Chandra* (Sk) which relates to the sun and the moon.

If we look at this Sanskrit understanding of *Dai Ko Myo,* we see that it relates to the *Bodhisattva's* Suryaprabha (sunlight) and Chandraprabha (moonlight). These two *Bodhisattvas* assist the Buddha of Healing: Baishajyaguru (the Medicine Buddha or Yakushi Buddha as he is known in Japanese).[47]

> *(Medicine Buddha/Baishajyaguru) ... became an important figure in later Chinese Buddhism.... the most common set of figures on the principal shrine in large Chinese monasteries consists of Shakyamuni[47] flanked by Amitabha to his right and Baishajyaguru to his left (which is symbolically the east, the direction in which the Pure Land of the Medicine Buddha is said to be located).* (Vessantara, 1998)[48]

As we can see, all the symbols are profoundly and extensively interrelated on so many levels. The genius of Usui was in distilling these complex ideas and philosophies into a set of simple symbols that could be used by anyone to help them sense the energies and for hands-on healing. There is a great deal more to be uncovered and learnt about the symbols.

Meditating on the Symbols

Now that we have some idea of what the symbols are all about, we should perhaps start to use them for what they were originally intended for: meditation.

> *The symbols have no power of their own – they act merely as a focus for a practitioner's intent. By focusing on a symbol or mantra a specific energy is stirred within the body.* (Stiene, 2005)[49]

This is really a moot point. In some senses it is true that the symbols are empty, having no power and reliant on the consciousness of the mind of the person that perceives them. If this were the only truth, however, it would mean that the symbols in Reiki could be anything; any design, any shape, and we could all just pick or make up our own symbols. Symbols and how they work are not as simple as this, however. In a sense, a symbol is a living, organic thing or entity. It has a consciousness of its own and acts as a release valve for psychic energy. If we look at the various associations that they have with different Buddhist deities, we can see that they very much stand in for the qualities associated with those deities.

Symbols link different aspects or qualities of reality together, so that when we focus deeply on them in meditation, energy is transformed and reunites the perceiver with the perceived. Different levels of reality are integrated. A symbol is not dependent on its visual or materialised form nor on its functional aspects, but on its spiritual attributes. It is true that a symbol requires the consciousness of the perceiver to come to bear on it, but in so doing, the symbol then unlocks the door to the knowledge that we are just a reflection of the celestial, primordial state of the universe; that the higher contains the meaning of the lower: that in duality is oneness and in oneness is duality. The symbols are filters that will attune you to a different level of consciousness.[50]

Rob Preece described this beautifully in his book *The Psychology of Buddhist Tantra* in relation to working with the deities, when he said:

> *The body is the vessel that contains the elemental forces of the unconscious, the emotions, the instincts, and their related psychological patterns and impulses. The use of… (symbols)… act as a catalyst for transformation. They provide the forces awakening within the body with a symbolic vehicle through which they can be channelled.* (Preece, 2006)[51]

Method

A good way to work with the symbols in meditation is to draw them out on a piece of A4 card, just as they were taught to you by your Reiki teacher. I haven't included the symbols in this present work out of respect for the request made to me by my Reiki teachers not to put them into the public domain. If you haven't taken Reiki training yet, no need to worry. You can still try out the practice. There are many versions of the symbols available in books and on the internet for you to use, though it would be better if you took Reiki training first and received the appropriate Reiki attunements/*reiju* (discussed in the next chapter). If you have started your training but haven't taken level 2 (or 3!) yet, then your engagement with the meditations will be limited by this lack. My advice is: go and take your second/third level as soon as you can.

Once you have the symbols on a piece of card, it might be a good idea to go over them with something like a silver or gold marker; something that will reflect light easily. Now place the symbol in front of you. Perhaps lean it up against your dressing table mirror or prop it against a wall. If possible, try to shine a light on the symbol so that it reflects the light. The rest of the room should be subdued, so if necessary, turn the lights down a little. Sit about three feet away from the symbol in your normal meditation posture and settle yourself.

Once you are settled, rest your gaze on the symbol; soften it by gently half closing your eyes. Now simply stay with the symbol. Your mind will wander, but just bring it back to its focus on the symbol. When you start to imagine and see shapes within the symbol just allow them to arise and pass away. You will imagine all sorts of things in the symbol: you might see eyes or faces or strange configurations that are just the mental projections of your mind. Whatever arises, just be with it and let it pass. It is very important to note that we are not making any judgments about the symbol or trying to see specific things or shapes or trying to "feel the energy." We are simply allowing whatever arises, to arise and pass on.

Once you have sat with the symbol for a few minutes,

try closing your eyes and bring the symbol to mind. Hold it mentally in front of your Third Eye. Again, we are just a neutral observer of whatever arises. We are not doing anything with the symbol or trying to see anything. We simply sit with it. If at any time you start to lose the sense of what the symbol looks like, you can always briefly open your eyes and look at the symbol in front of you again.

This approach to meditation will work well with Symbol 1 and Symbol 2, but what of Symbol 3 and 4? Symbol 3 is almost impossible to hold in your mind all in one go. It is very complex. What you can do is meditate on it in sections. You might want to focus on each *kanji* in turn, or maybe take two *kanji* together and focus on them before moving on. However, you should not do this all in one sitting. Stay with whatever you have selected as the subject for your meditation (let's say the first two *kanji*) for some days or weeks before moving on to the next one or two *kanji*.

You might like to consider meditating on Symbol 3 by focusing on the *Ze* as the central pivot of the symbol and then combining it with the other *kanji* in different orders. The *Hon Sha Ze Sho Nen* is a complex multifaceted symbol, and you can explore the depths of this more fully by changing the sequence of the *kanji* in meditation (so for instance: *Sho Ze* or *Nen Ze* or *Hon Ze*). It's important to understand the relationship of each character with the central *Ze*.

The following energy flow yantra shows the relationship of the various characters with *Ze*.

H
S Z N
S

Sho-Ze is an expression of the Ultimate Truth or the way to the Ultimate Truth (the true or correct origin. The true source).

Sha-Ze is an expression of supreme enlightenment (the true or correct person. One who has attained enlightenment). Thus *Sho-Ze* is indicating the path towards enlightenment and *Sha-Ze* is the result, the final integration of the mind and heart. This integrative state naturally leads to *Nen-Ze*: a true wish from the heart for universal compassion that arises as a consequence of the realization of the inter-connectedness and interdependence of all beings. This is the ultimate healing path. The final outcome of our journey through *Hon Sha Ze Sho Nen* is the realization at the core of our being that we are all one with the universal energy field. *Hon-Ze*.

With Symbol 4 you can if necessary, break it into smaller pieces to meditate on. If you can hold the whole thing in your mind all in one go, this is fine, but if not, try taking the *kanji* separately, just as you did with Symbol 3.

There are four symbols in the system of Reiki, but it is my belief that we should really be talking about two. Symbols 3 and 4 are not really symbols at all but *kanji* that express certain concepts and ideas expressed in the form of a *mantra*. However, they are still useful to engage with as meditation objects. If you wish to sound their *mantras* while you meditate on them, you can try this also (either out loud or quietly to yourself). Try it with and without the *mantra* and see if there is a difference. *Mantras* are most effective when intoned internally rather than being vocalized.

With these meditations, as I pointed out in relation to meditating on Symbol 3, you should spend some days or preferably weeks (or even months) with each symbol. Do not be in a hurry to move on to another symbol. Meditation is not a race, and the point of it is to simply sit and do it. See what, if anything, arises for you.

Sitting with these symbols is very much a *samatha* practice, designed to develop your powers of concentration and absorption into a single object or focus. As you engage with these meditations, however, do be aware of whatever else arises. Keep your mind open and aware. If your mind wanders, this is okay. Notice it, accept it and bring it back to the focus. Be mindful; be aware throughout these meditations. Don't try to "shut out" or force your mind to stop thinking. Allow whatever arises to simply arise.

Chapter 4

Bringing Depth and Balance to Your Reiki Practice

It's a natural human reaction to someone else's suffering to want to help them. However, this is not always easy and not always possible. If the suffering person is someone close to us, such as a mother or father, son or daughter, it can be excruciating when we find ourselves unable to help. We resonate on a deep level with their pain and feel helpless in the face of their suffering, which in turn can cause us to suffer along with them. Each twinge of pain, each mental or emotional relapse can set up feelings of guilt at our inadequacy in being unable to do something... doing anything that might help. If only we could minimise their suffering just a little and bring a sense of wellbeing and the knowledge that they are cared for. Sadly, one of the principal aspects of the human condition is the predisposition towards suffering. Another is the desire for the cessation of suffering in ourselves and for others.

A Reiki practitioner, drawn to the concept of healing out of an altruistic desire to help others, often developed as a result of empathy for the suffering of others, will often find that they are much more sensitive to that suffering than their non-Reiki friends. The critical factor that makes a difference between the Reiki person and the non-Reiki person, is the attunement (or more correctly, initiation) process that all Reiki practitioners must go through. Without an attunement you cannot practice Reiki.

Having its origins in esoteric Buddhist empowerments, an attunement is a mystical process that is at the heart of the whole Reiki experience; an initiation process that is performed by the Reiki teacher with or on his or her students. The modern-day

Reiki attunements are a development of a practice called *reiju* which was used by Mikao Usui with his students in the early years of the twentieth century. *Reiju* is still used in Japan and increasingly in the West, though the more commonly known attunement process is still dominant outside of Japan.

Attunements, Tandens and Chakras

The attunement or *reiju* impacts directly on the body's metaphysical energy system. Western attunements are generally understood to address the *chakra* system (energy vortexes, commonly referenced in Western New Age thought and derived from Hinduism and Buddhism[1]), while the original Japanese *reiju* is focused on the *tanden* system (energy reservoirs traditionally referenced in many aspects of Japanese culture and other Japanese energy disciplines such as Aikido).[2] The two systems are, however, simply different understandings and aspects of the body's energy matrix.[3] They are closely linked but they are not the same thing. *Chakras* are whirling energy junctures – transmitting and receiving stations, whereas the *tanden* is a reservoir or cauldron of energy. The attunement/*reiju* process is designed to elevate the body's energy and receptivity to universal energy, increase the vibration of various energy centers within the body and sensitise the practitioner to the flow of that energy. This is done by increasing the spin of various *chakras* thus raising their vibration to a higher state.

It has long been believed in the West that the attunement "gives" a student some special ability, but this isn't the case. In fact, it's an energetic reminder to the student of their own innate connectedness to all-that-is, to the oneness of the universe, in fact, to their own Buddha Nature. During this process the teacher and the student connect energetically and become one with the support of the attunement/*reiju*. In so doing, two consciousnesses merge to share the same experience of reality for a moment.[4] That experience is the dissolution of duality, a profound stillness and utter bliss.

When we practice Reiki as a healing modality or as a meditation practice, we once more reconnect to the true nature of the universe, to our True Nature. From the perspective of duality there is the experience of "flow" through an energy channel, and then through the *nadis*[5] (subtle streams or flows of energy within the body) created by the initiating Master from an external source: the universal energy field, but this is incorrect as there is no "external" in an absolute sense. Conceptually the understanding is useful, however, as it describes our real-life experience very well. Duality and oneness are, in fact, coexistent. We could say that what is happening when we experience a flow of energy at an energy center (*chakra* or *tanden*) is the mind observing the activity of the mind; mind is everywhere within and without the experience of being human.[6]

Experientially, from a Western Reiki perspective that is reliant on the *chakra* system, we can see that energy flows from the universal energy field, via *Sahasrara chakra* (crown) and makes use of the main *nadis* running along either side and within the spine: *Ida* (the left energy channel) *Pingala* (the right energy channel) and *Sushumna* (the central energy channel). In Chinese and Japanese medicine, these correspond to the *Penetrating Vessel*, *Conception Vessel* (*Yin*) and *Governing Vessel* (*Yang*) and lock us back in conceptually to the *tanden* system. The discussion over how the *chakra* system relates to the *tanden* system has been raging for centuries and probably will continue to do so. Suffice it to say that whatever system you were taught, it is best to stick with that and not try to combine it with other culturally different understandings. In the system of Reiki, working with either the *chakra* or the *tanden* system works just fine.

The *tanden* system is focused on an energy center just below the navel – called the *hara* or lower *tanden* (or lower elixir field[7]). There are, however, two other *tandens*: the middle and upper *tanden* (with specific *chakras* being a functional part of them), both of which are significantly impacted by the attunement/ *reiju* process. A good description of the middle *tanden* was given by Joseph Samsen and Heidi Hanson on their website, *The Gathering – Metaphysical Guidebook*. This *tanden* is related to our relationships with other people and is the location of the Heart chakra:

> *[T]he "middle" field of energetic elixirs (is) located in the center of the chest or heart center.... The middle elixir field is not simply the Heart chakra operating all by itself. The middle elixir field is a swirling, pulsating ball of energy created by the Heart chakra combining with lung meridians, prana from the environment taken in through deep breathing, the thymus gland, energies traveling up and down arms, in and out of fingertips or palms, etc. This "middle" field of elixirs is then clearly associated with the "middle" treasure of human experience. The chi energies. The way in which those energies related to relationships between things (beautifully symbolized by the way the arms and hands reach out from the chest for a hug) are in turn related to that place on the body where an equal "gathering" of... opposite energies takes place. An equal "gathering" of both Yin and Yang. An equal "gathering" of all those energies from the heavens above your head and the Earth below your feet. A swirling, pulsating "gathering place" in the center of your chest referred to by the ancient Chinese as the "middle" field of elixirs.* (Samsen and Hanson, n.d.)[8]

The upper *tanden* or elixir field is where our intuitive abilities and our insights into the true nature of the world around us begin to develop. This is the seat of the Third Eye. Reiki Master, Beth Hansen-Buth noted that the

> *Upper Hara (the Third Eye area, between and slightly above your eyebrows) relates to your upper chakras: Throat, Third Eye, &*

> *Crown. This is where you connect to your spirituality. Working with energy at the Heaven Ki level connects you to the oneness of all things, and your intuition guides you at this level.* (Hansen-Buth, 2007)[9]

A Reiki Practitioner can find quite quickly that their sensitivity to another's suffering is of a different order of magnitude to what they will have been familiar with prior to their attunement/*reiju*. This is due to focusing predominantly on the hands-on healing aspect of the practice (for themselves and other people), which, because of the attunement/*reiju* process, sensitises them intuitively and emotionally to whatever vibrations are around. This can develop the heart of compassion very powerfully and consequently empathic resonance can take a quantum leap. In instances such as these it is no longer a case of simply resonating with and understanding the pain of another from a far vantage point, it's more the case that the Reiki practitioner can experience that pain in a deep and personal way, right up close. It can be heartbreaking in a way that they have never experienced before, as they identify fully with the other person's pain, as if it were their own. One of my students, Nadine, sent me this message about what was happening to her because of her continued self-treatment with Reiki:

> *The more I practice Reiki, the more sensitive I'm getting to people's energies. I've been practicing on other people lately (and) it's great but at the same time I'm suffering. I can walk into a room of people, sit for half an hour, feel great as I am walking in and then leave feeling beat up like my heart hurts. I feel people's energy in my heart so I can tell if someone is hurting. I can tell in my heart. I recognize that it's not my pain. If I leave my house and go to the supermarket, it's becoming hard for me, so is there some way that I can protect myself?*

I should make clear that this sort of extreme reaction is uncommon, but it does happen often enough to make it worth addressing here. Even if you don't suffer to the same extent as Nadine, it's still worth taking the following points into account:

We need to look at the upper and middle *tandens* and more specifically at the Heart and Third Eye *chakras* within these larger cauldrons of energy. It's a given that one of the most important aspects of the practice of Reiki is the development of the heart of compassion. However, when this is combined with a highly developed intuitive ability without the guardianship of an equally developed state of balance and groundedness, we can be pulled very powerfully into the stream of suffering that another is experiencing. This does not help them, and it does not help us. We need to develop not only empathy and compassion, but also a mind of wisdom, and this is where we need to ensure we integrate meditation into our daily routine. It's through engaging in meditation that the flowering of genuine wisdom takes place. Wisdom is the key to providing both balance and groundedness to our Reiki practice so that we don't get pulled easily into another's suffering, as Nadine did.

Bringing balance to the three elixir fields will help to establish equanimity, stillness and equilibrium within the practitioner. To do that we must start from the base up at the lower *tanden* (*hara*). All things grow from the ground up: a tree needs solid, deeply embedded roots to sustain it as it grows upwards. A mountain has a firm base on which to sit. A human being is the same. We need to strengthen our connection to the lower *tanden* as well as develop the qualities associated with the other two *tandens*. Meditation on the breath (*anapanasati*), whilst focusing on the rise and fall of the abdomen, will take your awareness to the lower *tanden* and strengthen this elixir field. Developing a correct and stable balance between this *tanden* and the heart is critical. Laozi said:

> *Empty the heart, fill the abdomen.*[10]

So, before we get carried away with what the heart feels and start engaging in deep suffering with those around us, we need to sink our awareness down into our belly, into the *hara*... and be still.

> *[B]y centering our breathing entirely in the lower-abdomen or hara, the hara can come to be felt as a vast, warm and womb-like ocean of awareness – into which we can comfortably let our awareness sink or flow down into – yet without losing our center or sense of self.... This basic practice of centering both breathing and awareness in the warm and womb-like interiority of the hara is also the key to... 'belly thinking'.... For it is from the ocean of awareness that expands within the hara that all thoughts are first conceived and germinate....* (The New Yoga, n.d.)[11]

In a sense you could say that when you bring the mind back to the body and focus on the breath, you are bringing the mind back home. As we have seen, generally speaking, the mind is utterly missing the here and now while our body and breath just get on with their job, completely ignored by the mind. Meditation helps us to correct this imbalance. However, it's worth spending a moment looking at the relationship between the body, breath and mind a little more closely before we look further at the practice of meditation.

The Three Treasures

Prior to our birth, the body, breath and mind exist as an undifferentiated unity. This is the seed of our life prior to incarnation in this physical world: "the seed of life slumbering in the vast ground of the universe...." (Reid, 1998). In this form it is in its prenatal phase, which then transforms right at the moment of conception. It cuts off from and differentiates itself from the rest of the universe and takes on the characteristics of separation and individuality, like a drop of water separating from the ocean when a wave crashes on the shore. It is now a discrete conscious, breathing, separated being comprising of three principal attributes: body, breath and mind. As consciousness develops, it generally considers itself to be utterly separate from all the other separated drops that broke free from the ocean of oneness.

The mind of this human being is characterised by personality and ego and the belief (and embeddedness) in duality that separates him or her from all other beings. This person is capable of rational thought, learning and intuition. These characteristics of a human being are located in the upper elixir field in the center of the head. This field regulates the activities of the two elixir fields below it and is connected to the primordial essence of the universe above it. In Western cultures, we tend to put great store in the enhancement of the upper elixir field: the development of rational thought and scientific enquiry as well as intuitive knowing (Westerners with a New Age inclination are for ever going on about developing their Third Eye, without the vaguest idea of what that actually means) and forget about developing our core, down deep at the navel at our center of gravity.

According to Daniel Reid, the Three Treasures of essence, energy and spirit, which are located in the three elixir fields, are the subtle expressions of body, breath and mind.[12] They are not called the Three Treasures for no reason. They are our most precious assets, and should be looked after, respected and developed.

Mostly, people tend to wear their bodies out, abusing their physical being through lack of exercise, incorrect diet, smoking, drinking, drug abuse and all manner of other ways that deny the reality of the body as a sacred temple of the spirit. We breathe badly, high up into our chests instead of down into our abdomen, or we abuse our ability to breathe entirely by smoking, and whilst all of this physical abuse is going on, we project forward and backward in time with our minds. If we want to negate suffering, then we need to bring the three treasures of essence, energy and spirit together and work with them as a unified whole.

The Japanese Buddhist monk and founder of Shingon Buddhism, Kukai, wrote in *Attaining Buddhahood in this Body*:

Form mudras with your hands,
Recite mantras with your mouths,
And dwell in meditation with your minds.[13]

This is Kukai's formula for working with the Three Treasures leading to an experience of the bliss of oneness: the realisation of our True Self and the unfoldment of our Buddha Nature and the larger universe.

Let's look at these three injunctions of Kukai's in the context of Reiki. Reiki is not generally known for its use of *mudras*, but we do use the *Gassho mudra* at the start of a healing session prior to making a spiritual connection with another person through the placement of hands in a healing context. In a sense every movement of the hands in a healing session, from the initial *Gassho* onwards, is a movement from one healing *mudra* to another (and as Frans Stiene notes in his excellent *The Inner Heart of Reiki*, would also include the attunements/*reiju*[14]). These *mudras*/movements symbolically identify the practitioner with the universe and are called *Shin-mitsu* (the mystery of our body's action). This element of the practice is the part that most people find the easiest: put your hands on and let the energy flow.

Mantra is certainly something that is very obvious and dominant in the Reiki system. There are of course the *mantras* associated with the Reiki symbols (*shirushi*), and in the traditional Japanese lineages of Reiki, the chanting of the Precepts. Working with *mantra* is called *Ku-mitsu* (the mystery of one's speech). Very importantly for this aspect of the system is the breath. The concepts of energy and breath are intrinsically interwoven. There is no *mantra* (sound) without breath. Sound is the frequency; breath is the energy that realises that frequency. There is no energy without breath. Breath and energy are essentially the same thing. Here is an exercise that you can try that shows the relationship between energy and breath: make a fist and watch what your breath does. You probably held it, yes? That's because the breath is the vehicle that drove the energy into your fist and holding the breath locked it there. Now make another fist, and this time deliberately breath through it. What happened to the fist this time? It probably got soft and quite useless, yes? The breath softened the fist, as it does whenever there is tension in the body (physical and mental/emotional). So, the breath and energy are absolutely bound together in every sense. There are methods that can be used in Reiki healing sessions that use the breath, such as *Koki-Ho,*[15] and some Reiki lineages that use the breath to transmit energy in the attunements/*reiju*.

So now we come back to meditation, or *I-mitsu* (the mystery of one's mind). This part of the system of Reiki is the hardest to commit to, but it's critical. By practicing meditation, we bring the mind home to the breath and the body. It's the method for the generation of wisdom, leading to an awakening and realisation of our True Nature.

Master of secret, how to attain wisdom?
Know one's mind as it truly is.[16]

To know one's mind, is to practice mindfulness. To be fully aware. In the system of Reiki, certainly within the Japanese lineages, there are a handful of meditation practices such as *Joshin Kokyu Ho, Seishin Toitsu* and *Kenyoku Ho,*[17] (the latter being a sort of moving meditational practice) that are designed to help with this. There are elements of these that are similar in intent and focus to practices within the tradition of Reiki Jin Kei Do,[18] such as the movement of energy in a meditation practice called the Six Point Meditation (a simplification of one cycle of a much more complex tantric meditation called *Buddho*[19]), which we will return to later. There are no specific meditations within the Western traditions of Reiki, where Reiki is predominantly focused on the hands-on healing aspects of the system and often only pays lip service to its deeper expression as a profound personal spiritual development system.

Any of the above meditations will enhance and serve you well in your engagement with Reiki. But simply engaging with the practice without a high degree of awareness will not get you very far. And as we have seen, awareness needs to be developed at the same time as the ability to become deeply concentrated or absorbed into the object of the meditation (*samatha*).

The potential of the mind is unlimited. When we work with the body, breath and voice, we use the mind to regulate them. There is a symbiotic relationship between the mind, the body and the breath (voice) and when we can regulate these treasures of the body and breath through the use of the mind, then we also gain a better control of the mind itself, without consciously having to regulate anything. So, we attain a state of energetic harmony. Once we achieve this state, we can sense any problem before it occurs and correct it.

Christopher Markert in his wonderful book *Dan Tien: Your Secret Energy Center* told a story of a Zen monk who had reached the highest levels of consciousness. The monk was asked how he occupied his mind during the day and the monk answered: "When eating, I eat, when fetching water, I fetch water, and when I go to bed, I sleep" (Markert, 1998).[20] The mind of the monk was centered and aware and focused fully on whatever it was he was doing at that moment. It was not wandering about and projecting into the future or the past and allowing a stream of random thoughts to cloud his mind.

We need to focus our minds, focus on the breath and bring our minds to our center: into the *hara*/lower *tanden*. Then we will develop a degree of balance and calmness in our lives and help to hone our awareness.

When we do this, we become more stable. Meditation automatically creates stability, and so we are not pulled this way or that by the emotional tides of life. When we encounter another's suffering therefore, we do not find ourselves being sucked into that suffering, as if it were our own, as Nadine did.

After Nadine resumed her meditation practice, she was much more able to cope with the waves of suffering that emanated from others. She was able to maintain her balance and offer compassion and support that was appropriate, measured and proportionate. When we can do this, the mind of wisdom is starting to flower.

Joshin Kokyu-Ho

This is a traditional Japanese Reiki meditation that is becoming increasingly well known within the Reiki community outside of Japan. One of the main benefits of practicing this meditation is that it helps to improve your ability to channel Reiki energy. It also helps to keep you very grounded, and this is a good thing when it comes to your further spiritual development. This meditation strengthens the primary energy channel: *The Penetrating Vessel* (or *sushumna*) running down the spine. The way it is generally taught, however, is with scant regard for the need to really bring a high level of awareness and focus to the practice.

You can practice this meditation for maybe 10 or 15 minutes when you first start, but as time goes by, if you wish you can extend that time to whatever suits you. An hour of practice is perfectly fine.

This meditation is based on deep abdominal breathing,

rather than the very unhealthy practice of breathing high into the chest. This might be good if you are a dancer and need to keep your stomach flat, but pretty much terrible in all other instances. The Chinese classic of internal medicine, the *Tao Te Ching* noted:

> *Can you keep the soul always concentrated from straying? Can you regulate the breath and become soft and pliant like an infant?* (Translated by Ch'u Ta-Kao, 1904, Chapter 10)[21]

It's important to sink our breath down into our belly, so that the breath flows naturally and deeply from the pit of the stomach or the *hara*. Below the ribs is a large muscle called the diaphragm, and when we breathe in, the diaphragm opens out, broadening and flattening in the body, pushing down on the body's organs and making the belly swell outwards. When we breathe out, the diaphragm resumes its former shape, folding back upwards, under the ribs. The diaphragm does this to increase the capacity of the lungs. Retraining ourselves to consciously breathe with the diaphragm is a very healthy practice.

> *The diaphragm is the ideal workhorse in the art of proper breathing. It's truly amazing what a difference it makes to health and overall vitality.... Breathing with the diaphragm is the key technique in all forms of chi-gung, as well as in yoga, pranayama, and all practices where breathing plays a central role. The benefits of diaphragmic breathing extend far beyond the respiratory system, greatly enhancing the power of the circulatory system, balancing the nervous system, regulating the endocrine system, and providing a deep stimulating massage to all of the organs of the digestive system.* (Reid, 1998)[22]

So, let's begin *Joshin Kokyu-Ho*:

Get yourself into a comfortable position. You can, if you wish, sit cross-legged on the floor in a full or half lotus if that is comfortable, or you can use a meditation stool. It is also perfectly fine to sit on a chair if this works best for you. The important thing is to make sure that you are comfortable and stable in your posture. A stable posture encourages a stable mind. You may, if you wish, bring your hands together to form a Gassho mudra for a few moments, and fix your gaze on the floor in front of you. Take your awareness into your hands; into Gassho. Reflect on why we hold this mudra. What are you feeling when sat with your hands together in front of you, as if praying?

Now just take two or three slightly deeper breaths than normal and allow any tension in your body to go. Spend a few moments going over your body, releasing any tension that you may find on each out breath. Consciously be aware of any tension leaving your body as you breathe out. Bring your awareness to your hara and notice the way your belly rises and falls with each in and out breath for a few moments.

Bring your hands down into your lap, palms facing up, right hand resting on top of the left, thumbs connecting. This is Dhyana mudra[23] *which helps to deepen your concentration and bring about tranquillity of mind and a state of inner peace. If you prefer, you can simply allow your hands to rest comfortably on your knees. Now close your eyes. If you wish, you can connect the tongue to the palate just behind the upper teeth. This creates an energy circuit through the body called the "Microcosmic Orbit."*

Now bring your awareness to your breath, breathing in and out through your nose. Breathe in slightly deeper than normal, allowing your diaphragm to pull in the air and allowing the belly to expand outwards. Be careful not to breathe too deeply and hyperventilate.

Keep your awareness on your breath for a few moments. Be aware of the sensation of the breath at the nose and notice where else you feel it in your body. Do you notice it just at the nostrils, or in the throat, the chest, or further down in the belly? There is no correct way to feel it. Just be aware of where you notice the breath most strongly. Notice how the diaphragm relaxes on each out breath and expands again on each in breath.

If at any time your mind wanders, just acknowledge this and bring it back to the focus of the meditation. It may wander many times, and this is okay. Every time you notice that it has wandered is a moment of success: you are being aware!

As you breathe out, try to use your stomach as if it were a pump, driving out any unwanted air from the lungs. And then draw in another long, deep breath, right down into the stomach. Notice how this feels.

Just keep this breathing up for a few moments, noticing the sensations of air against the nostrils, the rise and fall of the belly as your diaphragm moves, whatever sensations are present, just allow them to be, noticing them without judgment.

Now have the intention of connecting to Reiki energy, using the breath as a vehicle to bring it in to the body. Visualise and have a strong sense that you are breathing in Reiki. Bring it all the way down into your hara. Feel the energy accumulating at your hara. Maintain your focus here as you continue to breathe in and out for a few moments. Notice any sensations of energy at the hara – inside your belly. If you do not notice anything, this is perfectly okay. Just be present with whatever is. Do not try to force or imagine something that is not real for you. Just acknowledge whatever you feel or do not feel at the hara.

Now visualise that the energy from your hara is expanding throughout your whole body. See it rise upwards through your torso, into your head and down your arms and into your hands and your fingers. See it also spreading down into your hips, your thighs, your knees, your lower legs and ankles and down into your feet and out to each of your toes. Feel and get a sense of your whole body filled with this energy radiating out from your core, from your hara. Do you feel any sensations anywhere, or are there any emotions arising? Just notice them and acknowledge their presence. There is no need to do anything with them.

Now see the energy radiating outwards from your body to the world beyond. See yourself sat at the center of this expanding field of energy, that is sweeping outwards and affecting everything in its path. Stay with this process for as long as you wish. Really get a sense of the energy from your hara spreading outwards and washing over everything and everyone in its path, going on to infinity. Do you feel anything? Do you sense any tingling anywhere in your body? Any feelings of warmth, or perhaps cold? What about your emotions? Just notice what is there without doing anything with it. Broaden out your perspective and have a gentle awareness of whatever arises for you. If you don't feel anything, if nothing arises, just be aware of that. Whatever you are feeling or whatever you are not feeling, is perfectly fine and the way it is meant to be for this moment in time.

Let us now gently bring this meditation to a close. Bring your awareness back into your body and just be present with it for a few moments. Notice how your body feels. Notice any sensations of energy in the hara or anywhere else in the body. Raise your hands back into Gassho mudra.

Bring your awareness to your hands. Two things coming together as one – this is the point of Gassho. Duality giving way to oneness. Breathe into this mudra for a few moments, then open your eyes and reconnect with your surroundings. Take a few moments just to reflect on your experience of this meditation and then slowly move your body. You may now get up and resume your normal daily activities.

How do you feel after completing *Joshin Kokyu-Ho*? Hopefully very calm, peaceful and centered, as well as energised. It's important when doing this meditation to really be *aware* of what you are doing. There is a specific sequence of physical and mental actions that you need to follow to complete this practice: Sit in your posture, raise your hands to *Gassho,* look at the floor, close your eyes, breathe in Reiki to the *hara,* expand it through your own body, expand it outwards to the rest of the universe, bring your hands into *Gassho* and finish. That is the way most books will pretty much describe the process to you: a dry run through the basic foundations of the practice. What is critical in all of this is the *mind,* however. The mind is everything. What you do with the mind during the practice is significant. It is perfectly possible to carry out all of the physical and mental instructions for completing this practice and think about what you are having for lunch. This is certainly a topic that is likely to come up, since you are sat focusing on your belly so much! This is incorrect, however. Try to keep your mind on the task of being aware of every moment of the meditation. It's important that you train your mind to be aware of whatever *is*. We are using the faculties and abilities of the upper elixir field to work with and transform the experience of the lower elixir field (the *hara*) and doing it all with acute and focused awareness.

Chapter 5

Broadening the Concept of Healing

If we want to have a deep engagement with the system of Reiki as a therapeutic method, then we need to develop our abilities in mindfulness meditation as much as we can.

Back in 2012 and 2014 the Indian mystic Sadhguru[1] appeared in two separate but related YouTube videos where he was asked why one should not do Reiki to avoid karma,[2] and "Why do you tell people not to do healing?"[3] The first (the Reiki/karma video) we can to some degree dismiss because the question posed to Sadhguru was inherently flawed and set up a premise that had nothing to do with Reiki. Had the question posed been based in fact, then Sadhguru's answer would be acceptable in that context. However, his comments in that video in relation to the concept of energy healing are worth noting and were expanded upon later in a video about why people should not get involved in the practice of energy healing in general. These two videos left the Reiki community aghast. Here was a very well respected, world-renowned spiritual teacher, apparently undermining the practice of so many Reiki practitioners and masters around the world. Having watched these videos a number of times, I have to say, I completely agree with Sadhguru's comments, and what he said in those videos is pretty much what I have been telling my students in Reiki classes for many years. His comments don't in any way contradict the basic philosophy and tenets of the Reiki system. This is what Sadhguru had to say:

> *(Energy healers) meddling with another person's life process without knowing the whole of it is irresponsible.... Any kind of meddling with other people's energies is very juvenile. It's coming out of a certain immaturity and a certain egoistic state of wanting*

> *to play God.... Any problem in the body or in the mind is coming up only as an indication of a deeper situation.... All chronic illnesses are like this. They're just indicators of a deeper problem which exists. If you erase the indicator, it will find expression in some other way. They are only erasing the effect. They are unable to remove the cause. Just manipulating energies and erasing the effect is not good for you in the deeper sense of life. And for many people, their disease is not a curse. All this healing is a very juvenile thing.* (Sadhguru, 2012/2014)

Sadhguru's comments go right to the core of the practice of Reiki as a healing modality. When I teach a Reiki class, I always make it clear to my students that I will not be teaching them how to be healers. I am not a healer and have no intention of ever becoming one, though I have been involved in and facilitated many healing processes. We cannot *give* someone Reiki. One of the core teachings of the system is that Reiki energy is *drawn in* by the recipient for their own healing needs and not *pushed in* by the practitioner. To call ourselves healers somehow implies that we are in charge of the healing process; that we are "doing" something. As we saw in Chapter 1, we need to get out of this "Doing Mode" and into a "Being Mode" when it comes to our practice of Reiki. When we can just "be" with the process we start to embody the true nature of the universe, we start to connect to the true nature of reality, and this can have a profound healing effect on those around us. All of this goes right to the root of what Sadhguru was saying. To call oneself a healer or a Reiki healer, is profoundly egotistical. Not even Jesus, as far as we know, referred to himself as a healer. A Reiki practitioner is not healing anyone and to claim to be doing so is very arrogant. This was summed up beautifully by Bodo Baginski and Shalila Sharamon in their book *Reiki Universal Life Energy*:

> *[D]o not be disappointed if your expectations are not fulfilled*

> *immediately. With Reiki, nothing is to be achieved by pure willpower. Our egos have to take second place instead, which is not bad for our development. As Reiki channels, we do not do the healing ourselves but are simply neutral observers and witnesses of events. For this reason, we should never disapprove of a patient's symptoms. It is not our task to fight against an illness but to pass on Reiki energy and await the results, which will always be the best ones possible.* (Baginski and Sharamon, 1988)[4]

As a Reiki practitioner, you have no way of knowing what the deeper problem may be or where it is located in the energetic matrix or physical body of the human being. Here is an example that I regularly give in my classes: Let's imagine someone comes to you with a lower back pain. You can see he is suffering, and out of compassion, you might feel your heart open and want to help by fixing his back problem for him. What you don't know is that your client has a very bad relationship with his boss at work. He is regularly chastised, overworked, suffers the brunt of his boss's anger and is generally given a hard time. This produces a lot of daily stress. Over time this stress has lodged in his shoulder muscles so that they are extremely tight and painful. Slowly that tension and stress has moved down his back and he now has a lower back pain. His problem is not with his lower back per se, but in his relationship with his boss. You don't know this (and maybe your client doesn't make the link between his work-related stress and back pain either), but the Reiki energy does. So, all your attempts to solve his problem for him by focusing on his lower back are at best misplaced. You may alleviate the pain a little, but you won't fix the problem at its cause unless you allow the energy to do what it needs to do: target his relationship with his boss.

Fortunately for your client, the energy does not in fact need your assistance and it will go to where it is needed regardless of your attempts to focus it where you think the problem is.

Your "Doing Mode" attempt to make the energy bring about your desired outcome will simply "slow down" or hamper the energy's ability to do what it needs to do. Like a reed in a stream, we can either go with the flow where it might lead, or we can resist and find that the stream will simply flow around us.

There are some who believe that they can access the information regarding the original cause of things intuitively, and so target the precise cause or location. Mostly this is an expression of ego, because mostly, they can't. The information pin-pointing the original cause is certainly "out there" in the universal energy field (UEF) and within the energetic matrix of the individual. This information, however, when accessed by the Reiki practitioner is filtered through the human mind and is subject to various influences: the perceptions of the ego, obscuration caused by our own imperfections, sensory data filtering as well as cultural, religious, and time-specific influences. This all renders the originally "pure" information as potentially inaccurate or entirely wrong. The majority of people, including energy healers and Reiki practitioners, do not have the spiritual connectivity or spiritual awareness to "read" this information accurately and to know that it is being corrupted by themselves. They act based on what they believe to be true but are in fact working on the basis of an obscured, filtered or corrupted version of the truth. Consequently, energy is manipulated, eradicated, replaced and basically messed about with, by people who simply do not know what they are doing. Even if some people are gifted with the ability to perceive on very subtle levels the exact location and original cause of a physical or mental/emotional problem, why take the chance? The energy, this powerful manifestation of the oneness of all existence, still knows best! Leave it up to the higher intelligence of the universe. Your participation on this level of the healing process is not needed. It would be true to say that in some senses, once your hands are on the client, the treatment process is really no longer any of your business.

In working with Reiki, we need to broaden our understanding of what we mean by "healing" and stop picking up bad habits and philosophies from other energy healing modalities. According to the Online Etymology Dictionary,[5] the verb "heal" is derived from the old English word *haelan* which means, amongst other things "to make whole." Sometimes to make whole is less to do with removing the problem and more about allowing the problem to simply unfold. Every experience we have in life, whether it be the circumstances of our life, an illness or some other physical issue that impacts on our life, is there for a reason. Nothing is the product of coincidence, accident or bad luck, because there simply are no coincidences, accidents or bad luck. Everything has a purpose. So, when we work in a healing context, to bring about wholeness we need to be mindful of the fact that everything is there for a reason. Everything is there to serve us in some way; to help us grow beyond our current condition.

A great spiritual teacher who suffers from Parkinson's disease once told me that healing was not so much about being rid of a debilitating condition but learning to live a meaningful and happy life within the context of that condition. This of course, takes a lot of courage. If we can change our relationship to our condition in this way, then the problem ceases to be a problem and becomes a trigger for personal growth and for beneficial outcomes to manifest in all sorts of ways. As a Reiki practitioner, would we want to deprive this person of the blessings that can flow from the circumstances of their life? Sometimes healing is not about destroying the problem but embracing or befriending the problem and learning to be the best that we can be within that context; accepting the totality of who we are.

There is a story about Padmasambhava, the great spiritual teacher who was pivotal in the establishment of Vajrayana Buddhism as the dominant religious philosophy in Tibet.

Padmasambhava is also known as the Tantric Buddha, and he completely transformed the religious, philosophical and cultural landscape of Tibet.

According to the story, King Trisong Detsen, the 38th king of the Yarlung dynasty and the first Emperor of Tibet (742–797) invited Śāntarakṣita, the abbot of Nalanda University to Tibet to help establish the teachings of the Buddha there. Śāntarakṣita started building the Samye monastery but was hindered by demonic forces. Padmasambhava was invited to Tibet to get rid of the demons. He did not, however, destroy the demons. Out of his great wisdom and compassion, Padmasambhava encouraged the demons to submit to the teachings of the Buddha, thus helping them on their journey to a spiritual awakening. This is in alignment with the tantric principles of not destroying negative forces but using them to fuel the journey towards a better and more whole state of being.

This story illustrates clearly the need to accept, embrace and show deep compassion for the negative states that exist in life, whether this be external circumstances or internal physical conditions. It is this acceptance and ability to embrace things just the way they are right now, that the system of Reiki is also built upon.

In Reiki therefore we engage with this alchemical process by not "ripping out" negative energy and replacing it with positive energy when working in a healing context. We encourage the transformation of the negative energy, the health issue or other life circumstance, to take on a more positive aspect; to use it as fuel to bring about a more whole state of being. To do this we need to step our conscious minds out of the way and allow that transformative process to unfold in whatever way it needs. We are not looking for solutions or making judgments about what needs to be fixed.

Whilst writing this chapter, one of my students posted a status on Facebook: "May God grant us the insight to understand the wisdom of our hardships." There is indeed wisdom in our hardships. Whatever we are going through in life is there to help us in some way; to provide us with an opportunity for further growth. It may not seem like it at the time. Often life can be very difficult, and suffering can be profound and deeply traumatic, but if we are gentle with ourselves and nurture ourselves with love and with care, we can turn even the worst of life's circumstances into a positive force. This is as much true for our Reiki clients as it is for ourselves. We do not know what God/the universe/the divine power (or indeed our clients or our own karma) has in store.

To assume we know how to fix a problem at its deepest pre-manifestation state and to assume we know what healing means is, as Sadhguru has clearly stated, "juvenile meddling." This is why Reiki is so dominant in the energy healing field. The system has a much more sophisticated understanding of health and healing than many other energy healing practices.

It's worth reflecting for a moment on what we mean by "negative energy" in a healing context. What we perceive as being negative, or a manifestation of negative energy, as traumatic or painful as it may be, is in fact also an opportunity for further growth. It's possible to see all of life's problems in this way, whether they be physical illnesses or the circumstances of our life. When we see that something is holding us back or causing us to suffer, we tend to compound that state of suffering through our point of view; our mind loads secondary suffering on top of the primary suffering. We will come back to this concept of primary and secondary suffering later but let us consider further this concept of negative and positive. If you are a farmer worried about your parched and dying crops, a day of rain seems like a blessing. If on the other hand, you are rushing to your office on the other side of the city, rain is the last thing you want. But rain is neither good nor bad. It simply is. And what's more, it's impermanent. Nothing has within it an innate quality of negativity or positivity. Everything simply *is*. We could decide to look at the circumstances of our life and the state of our physical health in the same way. Despite our suffering, despite our difficulties, we can also see these as essentially empty of positive or negative attributes. When we can do this, we free ourselves so that we can then impose upon our lives whatever understanding that we wish. We can, if we wish, view these conditions of our lives as opportunities for further growth. Of course, this is not always easy. Far from it.

This orientation to life and the lives of others also applies to when we are working with Reiki in a healing context. We need to let go of the need to judge another's circumstances as positive or negative, and just *be* with the process. We don't know what opportunities are being presented. We can acknowledge our clients' suffering, we can feel compassion and support them through their healing process of course, but we must still "be" with their process rather than meddle with it on the basis that we think we know best.

Sometimes the healing opportunities that arise out of suffering when we are working with Reiki can come in the form of being guided or gently pushed in a particular direction; to perhaps change one's diet or to take up some form of exercise. Reiki might even lead you to another therapy or a flash of insight might occur that enables growth and healing to take place. This is what happened when I first met Hala.

Hala came to me with a severe problem in her stomach. She had recently had surgery for a tumor and the scar ran all around her midriff. When I met her, her stomach was as tight as a drum. The skin was stretched painfully across her stomach and was rippled, as if there were multiple lumps of some kind buried just underneath the skin. She was in severe pain which stretched from her stomach all the way down into her groin. Her doctors had no explanation for this and could not offer her a solution that could help correct the problem. I gave her a

Reiki session which seemed to help alleviate the pain, however, over the coming days the pain returned. Hala came back for another session and again the pain subsided but returned later, though in a much less intense form. This went on for a number of sessions, but the pain was not going. Sometimes the pain got worse instead of lessening, but Hala put her trust in me and kept coming for her weekly Reiki sessions.

Then on our final session it suddenly occurred to me that the pain that Hala was experiencing might somehow be linked to her breathing. I asked her to stand up and show me how she breathed. Hala took a deep breath into her chest. "Why do you breathe like that?" I asked. "You should be breathing down into your stomach. Try breathing into your belly." She couldn't.

Most of us find that as we get older, our breathing rises to our chest, so that most adults believe that the chest muscles somehow control their breathing. This is very unhealthy and in Hala's case had been a conscious decision. She was a professional dancer, performing regularly at the Cairo Opera House and her dance instructor had told her to breathe high into her chest to keep her belly flat. If you're a dancer, you will understand this.

"There's your problem." I told Hala. I showed her how to breathe into her belly and she tried it without much success, so ingrained in her was the idea that she should breathe into her chest and keep her belly flat. But at least, with the help of Reiki, we had uncovered the problem. In that day's Reiki session, the whole of Hala's belly responded deeply to the energy. I could feel her belly easing and releasing under my hands and her stomach began to gurgle as it relaxed. All of the tension went out of it and the pain completely disappeared, never to return. Hala now knew what she needed to do to maintain her health. She went away to practice deep breathing into her belly.

Let's take a look at a meditation practice that can help with abdominal breathing. It is a modification of a classic *hara*-based meditation which uses the flow of energy as the object of the meditation.

Energy Gate Breathing

Let us begin by establishing our meditation posture and placing our hands in the form of the "cosmic mudra," or if you wish, you can simply place your hands palms-down on your legs or loosely in your lap. If you wish to place a cushion in your lap to rest your hands on, you can do this. It helps to keep the chest open and expansive. Now gently take your mind around your body and check that your posture is solid and stable. Make sure that your spine is straight, but not over-extended. Your spine should be resting in a natural S-shaped curve. If you are using a chair, make sure that you are not leaning against the back of it, unless you need the extra support, and that your feet are planted firmly on the floor. If you can't reach the floor, you may place a block or cushion there for your feet to sit on.

Make sure that your body is natural and relaxed. There should be no sense of straining.

Check that your shoulders are not tense. As you breathe out consciously allow any tension in the shoulders to slip away. You should feel a sense of openness in the chest. Check that your head is balanced gently, imagining that you are supporting the sky with the crown of your head. Now close your eyes or half close your eyes and let your gaze fall gently a few feet in front of you. There should be a sense of quiet dignity about your posture.

Now take three breaths, breathing in up the spine and breathing out over the head, as if it were a waterfall, and allow your awareness to descend to your abdomen. This will help you develop awareness of your spine, your posture and energy flow and sets in motion the energy of the microcosmic orbit[6] *which will assist you in remaining still, contemplative, alert and focused on the hara. Just stay with this for a few moments. If at any time during this meditation your mind wanders, this is okay. Just acknowledge this and bring it back to the breath. Use the breath as an anchor for your awareness every time your mind wanders, and then return it to the focus of the meditation.*

Allow your awareness to sink naturally into your abdominal area and keep your focus on your breath: going in and going out.

Now take your awareness to the top of your head; the Medicine Palace or "ni-wang-gung." Keep your attention here for a few moments and if you have second level Reiki, you may, if you wish, visualise Symbol 1 here. As you breathe in, visualise or get a sense of energy streaming in through this point at the crown of the head. You can visualise the energy as a golden or silver stream of light if you wish. Any visual imagery that works for you is perfectly fine. Notice any sensations manifesting here at the crown of the head. Go deep into those sensations and watch how they change, move and fluctuate. If you do not notice any sensations, this is okay, just keep your attention there for a few moments.

Now take this energy from the crown all the way down into the lower tanden, into the center of the hara, which is the elixir field, just below the navel. Guide this energy down with your breath. See the energy moving down and being stored in the hara. You may like to visualise Symbol 1 spiralling or flowing down to the hara. Again, use whatever visual imagery works for you. If at any point you feel strong sensations of energy as you guide it down, just stay with that for a few moments. Keep packing the energy into your hara and get a sense of what this feels like. You may use your breath to help you if you wish. The breath is a great vehicle for moving energy. Place your attention into your hara, into the elixir field, and have an awareness of any sensations there. Really go deep into this experience and stay there for a few moments.

Can you feel any sensations in any other part of your body? If so, just stay with them for a few moments. It is while cultivating energy from the hara that the emptiness of non-doing brings you peace and brings you back to your source, to your true nature.

Now move your awareness to your palms; to the Labor Palace or "lao-gung" and on each exhale, drive the energy from your hara up your spine and out to your palms. Visualise Symbol 1 flowing to your palms via the spine, from the hara. See it spinning and vibrating in each palm – a ball of energy.

On each inhale energy is manifesting at the Medicine Palace at the crown of your head and flowing down to the hara and on each exhale, it is now flowing from the hara to the hands. Feel the energy manifesting at the hands. Really go into that sensation of energy and notice how it feels; how the energy moves and changes and fluctuates. Stay with this for a few moments. Let your mind settle effortlessly in the hands. Let go of your focus on your breath and just allow it to flow to the hara on each inhale and to the hands on each exhale. Then allow your awareness to rest in your palms. Remember, if your mind wanders, simply notice this and bring it back to your breath and then to the focus.

Be aware of any sensations throughout your body. Notice the way the energy moves and manifests at our three points: the crown of the head, the hara and the palms of the hands.

If you are using this meditation during a treatment, you may like to cycle through it several times, or you may wish to extend the meditation to last the whole length of your treatment. When you are ready to finish gently bring your awareness back to your breath for a few moments. Expand your awareness back out into the room that you are in. Feel your connection to the Earth through your feet and in your own time you may open your eyes and end the meditation.

In some healing modalities there are methods that involve the removing of "negative energy." Some energy healers would say that this is what would seem to have been manifesting in Hala's stomach area. Had this negative energy removal been done, the root of the problem would most likely not have been uncovered and the pain could have returned at a later date, perhaps even worse than before as Hala would not have learnt the lesson that it was trying to teach her. By applying Reiki and allowing it to do whatever it needed to do, the root of the problem became clear and could then be addressed on the appropriate level.

Of course, as many who have worked with Reiki will testify, healing doesn't always come via direct solutions to physical problems but can manifest in the form of healing life situations or the circumstances of one's life. This can then impact quite deeply on the physical wellbeing of the individual.

A few years ago, I was working as a senior manager within the education sector in Cairo, Egypt. The place where I worked was, without a doubt, the worst organisation that I had ever worked for. There was nothing, not a thing, that functioned the way it should. It drove me crazy. At the same time, a friend of mine was working as the CEO of another educational institution on the other side of the city. I was for ever phoning her up and asking her if she had any jobs. I had worked for her before and we had an excellent working relationship. About six months into the academic year, she called me up and offered me the job of Vice Principal. I immediately said yes and handed in my resignation to my then current employer. I felt a huge sense of relief. All I had to do was run down the clock on the year and I was free; ready to start my new job on the other side of the city.

The day after the academic year ended, my friend phoned me up and informed me that the management team where she worked had just fired her. I was shocked. She was without a doubt one of the best bosses that I have ever had the pleasure of working for. She had been employed to turn around her organisation and make it into one of the best in the country. It wasn't failing, but neither was it going anywhere. It had settled into a state of humdrum mediocrity for the long term. To pull it out of this somnambulistic state required some effort and a lot of cash being spent. The management team, wanting to achieve their goals on the cheap, didn't like what their CEO was spending, and so fired her. You can do that in places like Egypt, and unless you're willing to go through the complexities and protracted paperwork of the local employment law, there is really little you can do about it. Especially if you're an expat.

I thought that my new job as the Vice Principal, however, was still secure. It wasn't at all. A few weeks later the same management team went down the list of all the new staff that had just been employed and wrote to them apologising for the fact that their services would no longer be required. I went into a panic. I had no job. I'd quit my old job and was unable to go back as someone had already been hired to replace me. It was the summer and if you've ever worked in the education sector you will know that this is the worst time of year to be job hunting. The last vacancies in the sector, across the whole country, had been filled some weeks before.

I spent about two months applying for every job that I could find. Only the dregs were left, but I applied anyway. I needed a job. I became very stressed and was starting to lose hope. I wasn't getting any responses of any kind to my applications, not even rejections. This was an entirely negative experience to my mind, and I wanted to fix it. I had bills to pay, my children to look after. Everything was black, black, black and I was in a constant state of panic, and my health was starting to suffer. Then one day, I just stopped.

"What was I doing?" I asked myself. I had spent a number of years wanting to get out of the education sector (many teachers will relate to this!), and finally, I was out. The universe had kicked me out the door, and here I was desperately trying to kick my way back in! I realised that I needed to re-orientate myself to my circumstances and look at it in a different way, through a different lens. In fact, this was not at all a negative situation but an amazing opportunity. Here I was without a job, but with many skills that I could turn into a new career. I'm a writer, an artist, a teacher of meditation, Reiki and Qigong and I had all that management experience. What was I panicking for? I could just work for myself.

I turned my back on my old career and refocused on the

career that was ahead. I started to promote my Reiki and meditation workshops in Egypt and started writing freelance for various English language magazines. For a few months, things were difficult, and I watched my bank account slowly empty. Then suddenly, just as my money was about to run out, my workshops went through the roof. Within 6 months, I had more students than I could possibly fit into the classes that I had scheduled. Through working with Reiki and meditating daily I found that, when the time was right, I was able to refocus my life and channel my energies in a new direction: one that was much more meaningful to me. As a consequence of this, although it was in some senses still quite a stressful time, I started to regain my balance and look at life in a much more optimistic way.

The lesson for me here was to learn to go with the flow; allow life's opportunities to emerge, and to trust in the process of life. This is exactly how we should approach our practice of Reiki: with trust, humility and allowing the wisdom of life's process to emerge; allowing to be whatever will be.

Byosen

How does all that I have said above impact on the Reiki healing method called *Byosen*? *Byosen* (or *Byosen Reikan-Ho* to give it its full name) is a Reiki technique practiced in the original Japanese traditions of Reiki which involves scanning the body for points of sickness where toxins may have accumulated. It's a method that also exists in the practices of Healing Qi Gong (though not under the name *Byosen*) and is not exclusive to Reiki.[7] The method involves identifying a place where there is clearly a physical problem by feeling the fluctuations and changes in the flow of energy from your hands and when it has subsided, moving on to the next *Byosen* point. According to Frank Petter, "The art of Byosen is neither intuitive nor psychic. Finding and following the Byosen is possible by becoming acutely perceptive and anyone can learn this" (Petter, 2012).[8]

So how do we practice *Byosen*, or indeed any method of giving someone a Reiki healing session, without getting in the way and potentially giving in to our egos and trying to manipulate or guide the energy and the outcome? Giving an effective Reiki healing session is very much about "being" and not "doing." It is critical that we should give up on what we think is the right outcome for the client and allow the energy to do what it needs to do. All we need to do is be empty; be still. It's actually really quite simple. As Jon Kabat-Zinn has noted, it's like climbing out of a raging current in a stream and watching from the bank.[9] In the quietness of meditation, our ego and its stake in particular outcomes gets set aside, allowing other alternatives to emerge. Frank Petter again:

> *Human consciousness becomes more powerful when it is empty of thoughts... you don't need an effort to give Reiki; it flows through you without your doing. Stop thinking while giving Reiki and become your hands. In this way, several things happen: First: more energy flows through you. Second: you don't get tired. Third, you are not tempted to have egoistic thoughts. Fourth, you discipline your mind while giving Reiki, and the treatment becomes a meditative experience of emptiness.* (Petter, 2012)[10]

Of course, as we have seen it is not possible to be completely empty of thoughts. It is possible to be effortless in how you conduct a Reiki treatment, however, and it is possible to eliminate the possibility of drifting into ego-driven ideas about what the outcome should or should not be. This is achieved by practicing mindfulness whilst giving a treatment. Once your hands are in place you can completely remove your consciousness from the treatment process by engaging in meditation. The practice of *Byosen* doesn't require your conscious involvement in any case. At its highest levels when deeply engaged in a meditation practice, *Byosen* can be given up to the energy. All you have to do is simply "allow" your hands and the energy will do the rest. As Petter said, when you can become "empty," more energy will flow, increasing the effectiveness of the treatment for the client.

The following *chakra*-based meditation can be used whilst giving someone a Reiki treatment. It works very well for getting your mind out of the way of the treatment process. You can also use the previous *hara*-based *Energy Gate Breathing* meditation in the same way. As both meditations use the flow of energy as the object of the meditation, this encourages a greater flow of energy for the benefit of the client as well as helping to develop your awareness and sensitivity to energy flow. You can also use these meditations as more formal practices. Just sit and do them as they are.

The following Six Point Meditation[11] is, like the previous one, a mindfulness practice that takes as its object of focus the flow of energy itself. It is regularly used in the context of giving someone a Reiki treatment and I routinely teach it from Reiki level 1 onwards. If you have access to the original *Buddho* meditation, from which the Six Point Meditation was derived, you will find the benefits in terms of your engagement with the energy and the treatment process itself to be considerably more pronounced.

Six Point Meditation

Let's start by establishing our meditation posture. Make sure that you are comfortable and that your hands are resting comfortably in your lap. You may wish to place a cushion in your lap to rest your hands on. This will help to keep the chest open and expansive rather than closing it up due to the downward drag of the weight of the arms and hands.

Take in a few slightly deeper breaths than normal and feel your body relaxing on each out breath. Feel your shoulders relaxing. Then allow your breath to return to normal. Gently take your mind around your body and check that your posture is stable, and you have a sense of being grounded. Check that your spine is straight and resting naturally. Your spine has a natural S-shape to it, so you do not want to be "ram-rod" straight. Rest into its natural curve. If sat on a chair, you might like to sit a little forward of the back of the chair unless you have lower back problems, then by all means, rest against the back of the chair or place a cushion there. Make sure that your feet are planted firmly on the floor. If you can't reach the floor, you may place a block or cushion there for your feet to sit on.

Check your shoulders. Let go of any tension on each exhalation. Check that your head is balanced. Imagine that you are supporting the sky with the top of your head. Now close your eyes or half close your eyes and let your gaze fall gently a few feet in front of you. There should be a sense of quiet dignity about your posture.

Bring your attention to your breath, going in and out. Notice where the process of breathing impacts on your body. Where do you feel it the most? Do you feel it at the nostrils or the chest? Or do you feel the rise and fall of your abdomen most strongly? Can you get a sense of the breath in the back of your body? Can you notice how the breath impacts on the whole of your physical being? It's like an ocean swell; rising and falling on each in and out breath. Just stay with the breath for a few moments.

If at any time during this meditation your mind wanders, this is okay. Just acknowledge this and bring it back to the breath. Use the breath as an anchor for your awareness every time your mind wanders, and then return it to the focus of the meditation.

Now take your awareness to the crown of your head, where we find the Crown chakra: Sahasrara. If you have second Degree Reiki, you may like to visualise Symbol 1 at the Crown, but this meditation works just fine without the symbol. Now place your awareness into the flow of energy at your Crown. Notice how it moves and changes. How it fluctuates. Really try to go deep into the sensation of energy at the Crown. If you don't notice any sensations, this is okay. Just keep your awareness at the Crown for a few moments. If you wish, you may visualise a stream of energy coming into your Crown from the Universal Energy Field. Try to get a sense of the feeling of energy at the Crown chakra. Stay with this for a few moments.

Now take your awareness down to the Third Eye chakra: Ajna. Again, if you have second Degree, you may place Symbol 1 at this point. Place your awareness into the experience of energy at the Third Eye. See how it moves and changes; how it fluctuates. Have a sense of the energy of the Universe coming in through the Crown and now down to the Third Eye. Really go deep into the sensation of energy at this chakra. Again, if you don't notice any sensations, this is fine. Just keep your awareness at the Third Eye for a few moments.

Now take your awareness down to your Throat chakra: Vishuddha. See the stream of energy from the Universe coming in through the Crown, down to the Third Eye and now down to the Throat. Place Symbol 1 there if you wish and are able to do so. Notice how the energy changes, moves and fluctuates. If you don't feel any sensations, just keep your awareness at the Throat for the time being. If you do feel the sensations of energy at the Throat, then try to go really deep into that experience if you can.

Take your awareness down to the Heart chakra: Anahata. Place Symbol 1 there if you wish. Be aware of the flow of energy from the Universal Energy Field coming in through your Crown chakra. through your Third Eye chakra, your Throat chakra and now down to your Heart chakra. Notice the sensations of energy at the Heart. Going deep into that experience – noticing how the energy changes, moves and fluctuates. Really feel yourself merging into that experience of energy at the Heart. If you don't notice any sensations, this is perfectly okay. Just stay at the Heart for a few moments.

Now from the Heart chakra, take your awareness up to your shoulders and down the nadi channel in your arms to your palms. Try to get a sense of the energy moving down your arms. You may wish to see Symbol 1 spiralling down the arms to the palms as you slowly take your awareness along the nadi channel. Then place your full awareness into your palms. Notice the energy moving and changing, increasing and flowing at your palms. You could see Symbol 1 spinning in all directions at once in the palms. Stay with this experience for a few moments.

Now just bring your awareness back to your breath. Notice your breathing. Breathing in and breathing out. Feel the effects of your breath within your body. Slowly bring your consciousness back into the room that you are in. Become aware of your physical body and your connection to the Earth. You may open your eyes in your own time when you are ready.

Energy based meditations conducted in the standing position are often very powerful and take advantage of something called "potential gradient." This determines the strength of the polar field in the human energy system between the *Yang* point at the crown and the *Yin* point at the soles of the feet. The greater the distance between these two poles, the more powerful is the flow of energy between them due to the strength of the potential gradient. The consequence of this is that the standing posture increases and accelerates the flow of energy and brings about a resonance between the subtle energy field of the human body and the macrocosmic force fields of nature and the universe. In a sitting posture the potential gradient is reduced as the perineum at the base of the spine serves as the *Yin* pole, thus reducing the potential gradient and so the energy is much gentler and softer – less dynamic.[12]

As a formal meditation practice, the Six Point Meditation should be done as described above, but if you are using it within a treatment context to get your consciousness out of the way of the process, then you should treat it as a cyclic meditation, and go back to the start at the Crown, once you have finished focusing on the palms.

Getting your mind out of the way of the treatment is a very powerful experience, both for you and your client. You will be amazed at how much more effective your treatments are when you can cut your consciousness out of the process. As much as you can, become an empty vessel. The more you can take this on board and get out of the way of what is going on under your hands the better for everyone, and most certainly your client!

Music

It's worth briefly mentioning the topic of using music during a treatment session at this point. Like many people involved in holistic therapies, I always used to put on some soothing New Age music whenever I had someone coming for a Reiki treatment. I never really gave it much thought. Everyone did it. I remember my Reiki Masters used to put music on or play Buddhist *mantras* in the background when I was taking my training with them. So, putting music on during a treatment was to me an intrinsic part of the process of giving a Reiki treatment.

When I moved to Egypt and started practicing Reiki there, I didn't have my collection of New Age CDs with me that I normally resorted to for treatment sessions. Playing The Doors or Pink Floyd or Leonard Cohen (which I did have with me!) in the background somehow didn't seem appropriate, so I left the room silent.

What happened as a consequence of this was that my meditation practice during the treatment process deepened and I felt a greater sense of stillness. This resulted in my clients getting a much better Reiki treatment. If you recall, I mentioned previously the playing of music during a formal meditation practice and how this is going to profoundly color and influence the quality of your meditation. The same thing applies when giving someone a Reiki treatment. Reiki is often referred to as "meditating with the hands," so perhaps we should start treating it as a meditative experience and turn the music off. It does interfere with the quality of your treatments quite dramatically.

One of my students made the point that in the health care setting where she works and offers Reiki treatments, her clients expect there to be soothing music in the background as it helps them relax. It's a good point but if you don't offer it in the first place, then they won't know to expect it. You are there to give them a quality healing experience with Reiki, not to entertain them. Reiki does the relaxation work; music is not required. Having suggested to my students that they try giving treatments without the New Age music playing, without exception they all reported an enhanced engagement with the energy and that their clients noticed a qualitative difference. The treatments were "much more powerful," they said.

In the end, whether working on yourself or working on someone else, Reiki is a spiritual practice, a spiritual experience. Working on someone else is really the same as working on yourself. If you want to explore the potential that Reiki has to offer, then just like when you sit to meditate, you really need to give yourself a fighting chance and turn the music off.

Chapter 6

How the Mind Relates to Suffering & What to Do About It

In the Pali language, the language of the Buddha, the word that is used to describe suffering is *dukkha*. We could also translate *dukkha* to mean "un-satisfactoriness" or "dis-ease." We know from our own experience of life that we are all prone to various kinds of suffering, un-satisfactoriness, aches, pains, illnesses and dis-eases of various kinds. The Buddha talked about our predisposition towards *dukkha* and what we could do about it in the Four Noble Truths[1] which is the main focus of what is widely believed to be the Buddha's very first teaching, given at the deer park near Benares in India immediately following his enlightenment. This teaching is recorded in the *Dhammacakkappavattana Sutta* (The Setting in Motion of the Wheel of the Dharma Sutta)[2] and was given to the five ascetics who had been the Buddha's former companions.

The Truth of Suffering (*dukkha*)

The Buddha made clear that all human beings are prone to *dukkha*. It doesn't matter if you are rich or poor, old or young; you are going to have pain and you are going to have suffering in your life. The roots of *dukkha* can come in any form: physical pain, emotional torment or as psychological problems. It doesn't matter how enlightened you get you cannot escape the roots of *dukkha*. Even the Buddha was prone to sickness.

> *When the Blessed One had entered upon the rainy season, there arose in him a severe illness, and sharp and deadly pains came upon him. And the Blessed One endured them mindfully, clearly comprehending and unperturbed.* (Sister Vajira & Story, 1998)[3]

We see here that the Buddha, although susceptible to the arising of sickness, was able through the practice of mindfulness to escape from his suffering. As much as we would like to banish suffering for ever, to consign it to the history books for the rest of eternity, this is not going to happen until, like the Buddha, we can bring mindfulness to our human frailty. Just as we solve the riddle of one virus, one disease, one dilemma, another potentially cataclysmic problem arises to be inflicted on humanity or upon our personal lives. As I write this the world is in the grip of the coronavirus pandemic and many people are suffering. This never-ending flow of bad times, illnesses, wars and epidemics will always remain an intrinsic part of the human condition. The truth of the suffering that arises out of our human condition was expounded upon in the Buddha's Second Noble Truth.

The Truth of the Cause of Suffering (*samudāya*)

The whole of our experience of life is governed by our sense of self. We create the concept of "me" from the condition of continuity, the illusion of permanence and then relate to it as if it were real. The direct cause of our suffering is ignorance or a lack of realisation of our own ephemeral existence. From this sense of self, desires and cravings for things and experiences and states of being or becoming arise. We may wish to be famous, or rich or well respected or deeply loved. We may wish to own this or that or try to avoid this or that. There are things we want and things that we don't want, things that we pull towards and things that we resist and pull away from. Here is the root cause of all our suffering. It exists entirely in the mind, however. The reality is that every single thing that we perceive as being permanent, stable and concrete is simply the constant flux of the universe in the process of becoming and ceasing. As Norman Fischer noted: "We think we can know and possess our lives, our loves, our identities, and even our possessions.

We can't" (Fischer, 2017).[4] And the reason for this is that there really is nothing to hold on to.

The Truth of the Cessation of Suffering (*nirodha*)

The Buddha made it clear that it is entirely possible to be free from suffering and if we truly wish to bring this suffering to an end, we must control our desires and practice non-attachment. We must stop grasping, pulling towards and pulling away from things. We must accept our reality as it is. This isn't to say that we stop caring about anything or that we stop setting goals for our lives. We can still dream and have ambitions, but we need to release our attachments to those dreams and ambitions and come from a place of profound acceptance and allowing of whatever arises, to simply arise. In this state we find that the friction that our desires habitually set up between our mind and reality is gone. Our mind can rest in its true state and flow naturally and gracefully into reality. When we can do this, we free our minds and achieve the state of satori. This is the beginning of the end of suffering.

The Truth of the Way to the Cessation of Suffering (*magga*)

The cessation of suffering in our lives is not going to come about through the practice of Reiki hands-on healing. Whilst hands-on healing is a wonderful tool to help bring us back into balance when we go astray, the end of suffering will arise on the back of the incorporation of the practice of mindfulness meditation into our lives. When we engage in this practice, which we can energetically support with hands-on healing so that we have a seamlessly integrated practice, we develop our ability to concentrate in a very powerful way and this can lead to an expansive level of insight and awareness into the true nature of reality. As we begin to accept the impermanence of life and all things, tranquillity arises. Ignorance is banished as we see clearly the emptiness of all conditioned phenomena and that everything is interdependent with every other thing. As these insights arise, we naturally tend to break the bonds and attachments to how we think or want our lives and the world around us to be. At this point we are liberated from everything that brings suffering into our lives and finally we can live in a state of peace and happiness. This was illustrated in the famous story of the woman Kisa Gotami who went to see the Buddha following the death of her child. In a state of extreme distress, she pleaded with the Buddha to bring her child back to life. The Buddha told the mother that he would do so on the condition that she bring him a mustard seed from a home that had never experienced death. The woman, filled with hope, searched everywhere but couldn't find such a home. She went back to the Buddha having realised the impermanent nature of everything and that death will eventually come to us all, and so she accepted the death of her child.[5]

As we saw in the previous chapter, it is often the case that something new can be learnt about the human condition from approaching our suffering from a different perspective: one that is inclusive of the experience of suffering rather than one that attempts to negate its existence. We need to embrace this experience for what it is rather than attempt to deny it, push it away or catastrophise about it. And this is, after all, the lesson of practicing Reiki.

Since it is in the mind that all suffering is born, it is in the mind that all healing must take place. Suffering is the result of how we respond to the circumstances of our lives, rather than being a product of the circumstances themselves. Certainly, if we are to ever free ourselves from our experience of suffering, we must take full responsibility for our own state of beingness and realise that we have choice in how we respond to everything. Nothing is fixed. Nothing is a given. Everything is unconditioned. We need to lead a balanced life from a point of stillness and acceptance of this unconditioned nature of existence and realise the pointlessness of finger pointing at things, circumstances and people as being somehow responsible for our state of suffering. Of course, they are not. The realisation of this on a personal level is critical to our mental wellbeing. Whilst we continue to blame others for our circumstances or the way that we feel, we can never truly be happy.

In *The Mindful Way through Depression*, Dr Mark Williams et al., described the human tendency towards creating our own suffering as a by-product of the way our survival mechanism has evolved.[6] Imagine a gazelle: adrenalin pumping through its system, running for its life with a cheetah in hot pursuit. The gazelle is quite naturally engaged in an act of self-preservation and it will do all that it can to escape the jaws of its pursuer. But once a member of the herd has been captured, the rest of the herd immediately resumes grazing and will often do so not very far from the locality of the now feasting predator as if nothing had happened. In that moment there is no danger. No need to do anything other than be present with the task at hand, which is to eat. Human beings on the other hand do not on the whole respond in this way. For us, there is an intermediate stage of processing that needs to be considered and it's one that we are largely unaware of even though we do it all the time. If we consider the facts of the situation (A), and our reaction to the situation (C), we can see that there is something missing: the act of interpretation (B). The gazelle on the other hand has gone from A to C with no interpretative stage in between. Predator chasing = run for your life. Predator not chasing = be calm and have lunch. It is this interpretative stage, evolved as a survival mechanism, that makes us distinct from other species and which compounds our suffering. Whilst the gazelle moves on to a new moment, the human being begins to extrapolate from the available data and catastrophise: the predator is still present and still might come after us. What if he alerts all of his friends to how tasty we are? Tomorrow we might be surrounded by hundreds of them! Whilst this act of interpretation and projection from the facts of the situation has many distinct advantages for our preservation individually and as a species, allowing us to plan ahead and ensure that we are not caught off-guard a second time, it also has many drawbacks. It causes immense and continuous suffering on a personal and collective level. This is suffering that the mind has invented.

We can say that there are in fact two types of suffering. There is primary suffering or primary pain which arises as a direct consequence of the situation that we find ourselves in and then there is secondary suffering which arises as a product of the mind and gets welded on to the primary suffering. For instance, if we were to have an accident and break a leg, it is obviously going to hurt. We can call this primary pain or primary suffering; the direct experience of the situation that we are in, manifesting as a series of signals to the brain from the damaged part of the body. There would be a similar response if we were experiencing a highly stressful or emotionally charged situation rather than a physical one. This could be, for instance, an impending redundancy or a relationship that is falling apart. These signals are the raw data or core elements of the experience. Once the brain receives this information, the mind kicks in and begins searching its filing system for all the other times we might have experienced a similar physical or emotional situation. The mind is attempting to find a solution. In doing so, it generates thoughts, feelings, emotions, and memories that it associates with that pain-experience. The two sets of data then become bonded together: the raw data and the mind-generated responses to that data. Once this happens, we often cannot tell which is which. What we may believe to be one solid experience of anguish is in fact a multi-layered composite of various kinds of primary and secondary information, interpretations, and extrapolations. It is clear then that the pain or hardship that we are experiencing is a synthesis of primary pain and secondary suffering.

Human beings are biologically hard-wired to suffer it seems. Neuroscientists will tell you that we have something called a "negativity bias"[7]; a survival mechanism that we have evolved over the past several million years. Our species has spent most of its existence wandering around the great plains of Africa in small groups. In this context, our negativity bias has served us very well and been the single most important factor in the survival of our species. We don't have sharp teeth and long claws to defend ourselves against predators on the hunt and we are pretty useless at outrunning them. What we do have is our negativity bias which, always hyper-alert, has enabled us to anticipate, analyze and avoid potential threats and impending danger. Our brains default to focusing on the negative as a matter of survival. It is no wonder therefore that when we switch on the TV to watch the news, it is full of negativity: wars, disasters, epidemics, earthquakes and the like. We are neurologically programmed to respond to life through the lens of our negativity bias.

Imagine being out and wandering the African plains when you spot a tree full of fruit. Before approaching the tree, your negativity bias kicks in. Maybe there is a predator hiding in the long grass. If there is, it would be wise to prioritise the situation and deal with it as best we can. At this point the mind gathers its data and begins to interpret and analyze. Should you run? Hunker down in the grass until the predator has gone? Freeze and hope it doesn't see you? Or maybe confront it and hope that you can chase it away? Very rapidly your mind analyzes the situation and quickly plays out the possible scenarios and the potential outcomes. Of course, none of these scenarios are real. They are mental projections, fabrications of the mind, existing as mere potentialities. It may be, of course, that whatever strategy you decide upon – perhaps distracting or leading the predator away so that you don't get eaten, you don't in the end get the fruit. But you can always come back for it tomorrow. If the fruit is your priority, however, and you ignore the threat that is about to pounce on you, you may never get the fruit at all and in all likelihood, there won't be a tomorrow, at least for you. This is why our minds have become honed to a laser sharp precision when it comes to noticing and focusing on the threats that life throws at us, both from the external situations of our lives and from the internal currents of our own physical or mental/emotional pain, and we apply this with highly penetrating awareness. According to neuroscientists, it takes only a tenth of a second to notice a threat, but many times longer to notice something pleasant.[8] Our initial reaction to a threat is to file the information related to the experience in our memory for rapid recall should the need arise at any time in the future. Any positive experiences that we might have take much longer to embed themselves.

Whenever we experience danger of any kind, we have an immediate reaction when the amygdala in the center of the brain is fired up and powerful stress hormones flood the system: adrenalin, cortisol and norepinephrine. The amygdala is an almond shaped structure that has been called "the alarm bell of the brain." This is the control panel for the negativity bias, and it uses about two thirds of its neurons to look for danger or any kind of negativity. Once it has been triggered, we are in the fight, flight or freeze mode, any of which could give us a survival edge. When there is no predator or dangerous situation to confront, and we are feeling relaxed and calm, oxytocin is released. This is sometimes called the "cuddle hormone" and has a profound healing effect on the human system. The amygdala is a very primitive part of the brain and it makes no distinction between a lion in the grass about to pounce and our boss yelling at us for missing a deadline. To the amygdala, both are threats and so the negativity bias is fired up regardless. A good way of viewing our predisposition towards the negativity bias was described by neuropsychologist, Dr Rick Hanson. He noted that the human brain acts like it has "Velcro for negative experiences (attaching very easily) and Teflon for positive ones (simply sliding away)."[9]

In the modern world, it is not likely that we will need to worry about predators as we reach for a bunch of bananas in the supermarket. Our negativity bias will certainly have a significant influence over our daily lives in many more contemporary situations, however. If someone insults us or criticises us at work, we are likely to spend quite some time thinking about this one incident rather than the many compliments that we might also have received that day. If we read the news on the internet or in a newspaper, we are more likely to remember and think about the negative stories than the positive ones. Even if we have a day filled with positive experiences and one small thing goes wrong, our negativity bias will focus in on that one bad thing rather than the many good things.[10]

It is clear that our negativity bias has a profound impact on our lives in many ways; helping us stay out of danger but also leading us into creating stressful narratives and situations for ourselves where in reality none exist, and then responding to them as if they do. This is an automatic response to the circumstances that we find ourselves in, and not something that is generally under our conscious control. To bring some balance back into our lives, we need to bring conscious awareness to the negativity bias which will help to soften and sometimes where appropriate, even to negate its influence. This does not mean, however, that we are taking control of it and using it to suppress our problems. As Rob Preece noted in *The Psychology of Buddhist Tantra*:

> *Repression tends to drive these forces into an unconscious shadow, but they do not vanish. What we have actively held down*

eventually re-emerges as sickness and disease, either psychological or physical. When the energy of the instincts and emotions is not acknowledged, integrated, or transformed, it consistently buries itself in the organs of the body. This can result in all manner of illnesses, neurotic habits, and emotional patterns, reflecting a lack of integration of the energy therein. (Preece, 2006)[11]

It is critical that we avoid the creation of this unconscious shadow. Our emotional state depends very much on our interpretation of a situation. In a stressful or painful situation when the negativity bias kicks in, the mind starts building a narrative.[12] The story that it creates will fit with the known facts however fictional or absurd it might be. Once there, this story is very difficult to deconstruct. This narrative can have very powerful effects on our emotional wellbeing and if we try to suppress it or deny it, we create an unconscious shadow that can have a debilitating effect on our health and wellbeing. As a personal self-healing discipline, the practice of Reiki must require us to look at our own predisposition towards suffering and to deal with the situation as best we can. We cannot turn off the negativity bias (and nor should we want to), but we can bring balance and harmony into our lives by recalibrating our relationship with the negativity bias, which is to say, developing the right view and relationship with our pain, in whatever form it may arise. We need to actively embrace our suffering and befriend it. We need to *lean into it* as I was told by my meditation teacher. As we saw in the previous chapter, the art of Reiki, both as a meditational practice and as an energy-based healing method is about acceptance and the enfolding of pain and the struggles of life, to allow them to be transformed at the appropriate time, when what it has to teach us has been learnt. Sogyal Rinpoche put it this way:

Whatever you do, do not shut off your pain; accept your pain and

> *remain vulnerable. However desperate you become, accept your pain as it is, because it is in fact trying to hand you a priceless gift – the chance of discovering through practice, what lies behind sorrow.* (Baker, 1997)[13]

As we have seen, lasting happiness simply cannot arise if we are engaged in denying or suppressing the circumstances that we find ourselves in. Likewise, we cannot find happiness through attempting to "rip out" what we perceive to be "negativity" (as happens with some of the more unsophisticated energy healing disciplines). Happiness is on the other side of the veil of suffering. It may be obscured by our negativity bias, but it is there to be found if we are willing to search for it and be gentle with whatever we find. But we need to avoid simply being positive as this isn't going to work. Much of the positive thinking literature encourages us to do just that but this simply promotes and entrenches a denial of our true state of being.

> *[W]e might have decided that from now on we are going to be positive and have only positive thoughts... if we have only positive thoughts, we will be happy, and the world will love us. Having bought into this paradigm, we might sit down to meditate and prepare ourselves for an uninterrupted flow of lovely happy thoughts. And what happens? Reality strikes and our whole endeavour is derailed as we suddenly find ourselves getting angry about the barking of the neighbour's dog.* (Nairn, et al., 2019)[14]

The "think happy thoughts" approach is predicated on the basis that if we simply look the other way and focus on the positive then the negative will simply melt away of its own accord. It's an approach that assumes that the negativity we are experiencing is the cause of our problems when in fact it is an effect or an outcome of our problems. By suppressing or denying the existence of the effect we will probably strengthen it and then we will have no hope of uncovering the cause or if we already know what the cause is, of resolving it. The various ways in which we suffer are deeply rooted in our past actions and the events that we experience in life. These actions and events give rise to reactions and patterns of thought and behavior that in turn gives rise to suffering on many levels. The negativity bias focuses on and amplifies the negatives that we experience in life, which in turn creates secondary suffering as it gives rise to the process of catastrophising or the process of suppression or denial and turning away, that the "think positive" approach promotes. Because we are relinquishing ownership of the negatives in our lives, we can end up projecting our pain and other issues on to external factors or other people and blaming them for our state of misery and pain; fully abdicating responsibility for our own state of being. The way to get balanced in all of this and take full responsibility for our state of beingness is through the practice of mindfulness meditation.

> *By turning toward discomfort and unpleasantness and by intentionally embracing them in awareness when they do arise, we are expanding the heart qualities of openness and goodwill in ourselves. By cultivating awareness in this way, we are weakening our tendency to avoid internal experiences we don't like.* (Williams, et al., 2007)[15]

Committing to a practice of mindfulness will help us to reclaim our original state of health, which in an ultimate sense is the supreme state of enlightenment, because life is much more than just the absence of suffering. With the practice of mindfulness meditation, we can begin to explore the sensations or feelings of pain or stress or other issues that we might find impacting or lodged within the body in a safe space. Neuroscientist Fadel Zeidan investigated the ability of mindfulness meditation to soften the mind's perception of physical pain in a study carried out at Wake Forest University School of Medicine in the USA. This was done by scanning and then mapping brain activity.[16] Zeidan showed quite clearly that mindfulness meditation produces greater pain relief and simultaneously activates higher order brain regions such as the orbitofrontal and cingulate cortices.[17] Mindfulness therefore reduces pain through some very unique mechanisms and was shown in the study group to reduce the intensity of the pain by up to 40 percent. The more experienced the meditator, the greater the reduction in pain and unpleasantness. Mindfulness meditation, according to Zeidan's studies, produces a pain relief response that is significantly more pronounced than the application of standard doses of morphine or other pain relieving drugs.[18] Likewise, it has been shown that a regular mindfulness practice for those suffering from clinical depression leads to "enduring positive outcomes in terms of relapse or recurrence, residual depressive symptoms, and quality of life" (Kuyken et al., 2015).[19]

What is being described here is the diminishing of suffering as a consequence of bringing the mind and its awareness to the experience of pain, either physical or mental/emotional. Bringing the mind to the primary pain not only softens our experience of that pain but helps us to see the stark reality of that experience once the catalysing effect of the mind's creation of secondary suffering is removed. Being in the moment with the experience of the primary pain stops the mind from reflecting on the accumulated sensory data, imaginary projections into the future and memories of the past that it habitually uses to create the layer of secondary suffering. Looking at our pain in this way can often be an extremely uncomfortable experience.

Whenever we experience discomfort, stress or physical pain we can, as I indicated earlier, learn to "lean into" that experience without judgment and without labeling. The art of being aware is simply that: to be aware of what is and to see clearly the nature of reality, including our own pain, stress or other physical discomfort without the influence of the negativity bias. When we lean into our pain, we can find that what we thought of as pain or discomfort may well reveal itself to be some other sensation or some other experience. Perhaps the pain or ache or sensation has a tingling or a pins and needles quality about it, or perhaps a dullness of some kind. We might find that the pain seems to come and go, sometimes in very fluid and subtle ways, and at other times quite abruptly and dramatically. We might experience piercing explosions of pain, or there could be sensations of hotness or coldness. Sometimes the pain might turn into an ache or a throb. When we bring our awareness to the ever-changing nature of our pain experience, we start to see how impermanent these sensations are and that they can morph one into another and then disappear quite rapidly as they give way to the next sensation. This experience can be a little like watching clouds drift across the sky. If we imagine our minds as being like the pristine vastness of the empty blue sky, then our experiences of pain and other sensations and even our thoughts about our pain are like the clouds. Sometimes they can completely obscure the sky and at other times they can appear less heavy and oppressive. But either way, clouds never impact on the purity and expansiveness of the sky itself. Likewise, our experiences of aches and pains or emotional traumas, or our thoughts about these experiences cannot impact on the pristine purity of the mind.

As we begin to see that our experiences of physical, mental or emotional pain are like the clouds, impermanent and forever changing from one form to another, it becomes clear that they are not just one vast block of solid, immoveable discomfort, agony or anguish as perhaps we had first imagined. We can become very quickly aware that the only pain that really exists in our experience is the one that we are experiencing right now in this very moment. All the other pain is simply the construct of the mind. We can also see that it is possible to explore the nature of that real and in-the-moment pain and discover nuances and qualities within it that perhaps we were previously not aware of.

Uniquely for Reiki practitioners, this process of bringing the mind to locations of physical or mental/emotional pain will also result in the rapid flow of healing energy. The Six Point Meditation that was introduced previously can be used as a self-healing mechanism. If you are suffering from a health issue of some kind, you might like to try the following, but please do so in consultation with your normal health-care provider:

A Short Meditation on Pain or Negative Mind-States

Simply do the Six Point Meditation as was previously described and then take your awareness to the site of whatever pain you may be experiencing and hold your awareness there. If it is a mental or emotional problem, try to locate where it impacts or has an effect on the physical body. It is important that you do not drop into "healer-mode" and start trying to do something. Simply be with the experience. You may wish to place Symbol 1 at the site of the pain to accelerate or intensify the process, but otherwise simply stay with the experience. Lean into the experience and explore it through the lens of detached curiosity. Place your awareness into the interaction between the energy and the physical sensations of your body or the mental or emotional pains that you may be experiencing. Just stay with that experience for a few moments. Try to really get a sense of how the experience feels, right in this very moment. Next try to take your awareness to something pleasant in your experience.

It is extremely easy to find oneself constantly drowning in the experience of the negative. By bringing awareness to the positive or pleasant that manifests in our lives as well as the negative, we can develop a more balanced and straightforward relationship with our physical or emotional pain. Vidyamala Burch noted in *Living Well with Pain and Illness* that human experience includes not only pain and physical limitation but also much that is subtle and beautiful and that when we try to block out pain, we also block out love, tenderness and sensitivity.[20] Life is indeed bittersweet. It is a delicate mixture of the wonderful and the awful. When we can accept this and turn our attention to all that life holds then we can live a life that is more relaxed and open. Bringing awareness to all that life is can sometimes result in unexpected outcomes.

A couple of years ago I was suffering with an acute pain in my left knee that was causing me a lot of problems when walking. This was very frustrating because I walk a lot, sometimes several miles in a day. I decided to explore the pain through meditation and lean into it and find out just what it had to tell me. To begin with I was quite nervous about this. I did not actually want to confront the pain. I just wanted it to go away and the thought of exploring it in meditation was quite unnerving. I expected the pain to intensify while my mind was consciously exploring it, so I approached the practice with some trepidation. For a week or more I sat and brought my mind to focus on the pain in my leg. As the practice went on, I began to understand the subtle nuances of the pain that I was experiencing, which dutifully throbbed and seemed to become more pronounced whilst my mind was focused on it. I was very aware of a flow of energy to the site of this pain. This caused a tingling sensation and an energetic heat seemed to be layered up on top of the heat that was generated by the pain itself. This was a strange sensation but the two "heats" were certainly of different qualities. Whilst it had my attention the pain seemed to be shouting at me even louder than normal. Then one day in the middle of a regular meditation, I suddenly had a flash of insight into the nature of what I was experiencing at my knee. A great big chunk of the pain suddenly morphed into something else; an entirely different sensation that wasn't pain at all. In fact, it had never been pain in the first place. At the very same moment a memory of my childhood popped up of a time when I had experienced the exact same sensation previously. It was as if my mind was saying "It's not pain, it's this" and pointing to the childhood memory for me to get an understanding of exactly what it was that I was experiencing. I was completely stunned. Right there in the middle of the meditation my whole orientation to my experience of what had been at times excruciating pain suddenly changed. When I realised that so much of what I had thought of as pain had been completely fabricated by my own mind, it instantly dropped away, and my level of suffering just melted like snow in springtime.

Our ability to face the inevitability of pain and dissolve our self-imposed suffering was illustrated in the following text from the *Sallatha Sutta* (often referred to as the "Arrow Sutra"):

> *Now the well-instructed disciple of the noble ones, when touched with a feeling of pain, does not sorrow, grieve, or lament, does not beat his breast or become distraught. So, he feels one pain: physical, but not mental. Just as if they were to shoot a man with an arrow and, right afterward, did not shoot him with another one, so that he would feel the pain of only one arrow. In the same way, when touched with a feeling of pain, the well-instructed disciple of the noble ones does not sorrow, grieve or lament, does not beat his breast or become distraught. He feels one pain: physical but not mental.* (Dinsdale, 2010)[21]

The first arrow is our primary pain: that aspect of our experience that we can do little about (like the pain that I had in my knee). The second arrow is the suffering that the mind has layered up on top of the primary pain. If we can learn to be the "well instructed disciple of the noble ones" we can, through our own conscious awareness experience just one arrow.

As we can see, it is our own resistance, catastrophising, denial and interpretation of our pain that causes us to suffer. This can often manifest in the form of stress which is the root cause of many of our physical and mental health issues. The word "stress" was brought to prominence by Dr Hans Selye in the 1950s in relation to his studies in animal behavior. He defined it as "the nonspecific response of the organism to any pressure or demand."[22] Stress therefore is the consequence of how we react to pressures or pains or external situations that we read through the lens of our negativity bias. This stress can have a major and direct impact on our immune system, making us more vulnerable to disease. The American Medical Association says that stress is implicated in up to 90 percent of all visits to a doctor.[23] This is a truly appalling statistic and reflected similarly in other countries. Practicing mindfulness meditation can help to significantly reduce the incidence of stress in the world and thus the incidence of other stress-related health issues.

Thoughts and What to Do About Them

One thing that we should be vigilant about is falling into the trap of thinking *about* our issues rather than exploring them from the "inside." What we are trying to do in our practice is to get in touch with and become deeply immersed in the experience of life unfolding, moment by moment, rather than simply thinking about life. In developing this capacity, our own body is a great place to start. The human body provides a great deal of sensory data that allows us to develop a powerful experiential way of knowing the world. Our bodies are always with us, so we have the perfect opportunity at any moment to bring our mind into contact with direct experience. Dr Mark Williams et al. gave the following simple experiment to illustrate the point.[24]

Start by closing your eyes and think about your hands; either both at the same time or one or the other. It doesn't much matter. You will probably have in mind an idea of how your hands look from the perspective of your eyes. We all know what our hands look like and where they are located on our body, but we are separate from them. We may think our hands are ugly, too fat, too skinny, have fingers that are too long or too short, or we might think our hands are beautiful or strong or maybe weak. We can have lots of thoughts about our hands, from the 'outside'. Now let's approach our hands from a different perspective.

With your eyes still closed, take your mind right inside your hands. Feel down deep into the fingers and the fingertips, the palm of the hand, around its edges, the knuckles. Get a sense of what that feels like from the inside. Perhaps you can notice some tingling or some warmth or an ache or pain somewhere. Maybe a tightness or a sense of relaxation. These are experiences from inside of the hand that are not 'hand-shaped'. What we are experiencing is a pattern of sensory data. So, it's important to bring our mind to our body in the right way.

An excellent practice to develop our skills of experiencing the body directly rather than thinking about the body is the Body Scan meditation. The Japanese approach to the Body Scan given here is always to start at the top of the head and work down towards the feet. This is to encourage a sense of being solid on the earth and for grounding.

The Body Scan

One of the benefits of the Body Scan is the powerful integration of mind and body that it provides whilst keeping the mind moving. Certainly, for beginners this constant flow of movement can be easier than trying to focus for long periods on a single focus-point. You can do this meditation either standing, sitting or lying down. There is a Japanese proverb that says, "the reclining person can't fall over," so with this in mind, the following instructions assume that you are lying down. If you are doing the meditation in some other posture, then please adapt the instructions accordingly. The following meditation is a variation of the one given by Julian Skinner and Sarah Bladen in their book *Practical Zen for Health, Wealth and Mindfulness*.[25]

Let's start by establishing our meditation posture. Make sure that you are comfortable either lying on your back or on your side. Make sure that your spine is straight but resting naturally so as to express its normal S-shaped curve. Place a cushion under your head so that your neck is neither compacted, or overly stretched at the back or front if you are lying on your back, or at either side if you are lying on your side. Have your legs outstretched but if this causes you any pain or discomfort you can place cushions under your knees so that you are lying in the semi-supine position. Your arms can either be resting at the sides of your body, palms up, or placed gently on your abdomen. Close your eyes or you may have them half-open and place your tongue at the roof of your mouth.

Now gently give yourself up to gravity. Really allow yourself to sink down into a fully relaxed state, feeling your weight held by the force of gravity. Allow your breathing to relax. Feel deep relaxation entering your body on each out breath. Let yourself go, more and more. Now place your attention on your abdominal area, at your lower tanden. Be aware of the rise and fall of the belly on each in and out breath. What can you feel here? Be sensitive to whatever may arise. Stay with this for a few moments.

Now bring your attention to the crown of your head and notice what you feel there. If you feel a flow of energy, this is fine. If not, this is also fine. Don't try to make anything happen, just be with whatever you experience at the crown. If your mind wanders this is okay, just bring it back to your crown as soon as you notice.

Whenever your mind wanders, this is perfectly okay. Simply accept that this is the normal process of the conditioned mind. Just note where the mind has gone and bring it back to the focus of the meditation. Each time you are aware of your mind having wandered, is a moment of success.

Now bring your awareness to your forehead. If there is any sense of tension here, notice how this softens as you bring your awareness to it. Take your awareness around to the side of your head above your ear and then to the back of your head opposite your forehead, then to the other side of your head above your ear.

Take your awareness to your eyes. Again, if there is any tension here, feel them naturally relax and soften with your mind's gentle focus upon them. Move your awareness around to your ear, then the back of your head and then the other ear. Move your awareness to your nose. Be aware of any sensations at your nose, especially the movement of the breath. The in breath and the out breath.

Move to your mouth. Move your awareness around your lips, first the upper lip and then the lower lip. How do they feel? Move to the jaw on one side of the head, then to the back of your head at the base of the skull and then finally the jaw on the other side of the head. Now move down to your throat and to one side of your neck. It doesn't matter which side. Move from here to the back of your neck and then to the other side of your neck. Keep bringing your mind back each time it wanders.

Move down to your chest, noticing how this feels first on one side, perhaps over the heart and then on the other side. Then moving under your arm and around to your back and then under the other arm, emerging again at the chest area. Noticing your upper arms, first one and then the other. Now back to your chest and the solar plexus area. Taking your awareness around to the side of your body, the back of your body at this height and then the other side of your body.

Take your awareness down to your abdomen, and to the side of your abdomen, the back of your body at the height of your abdomen and then the other side of the body. Noticing your elbows on each arm. Then taking your awareness down to your navel area. Being aware of this area before moving on to one side of the body at this level, and then the back of the body and the other side of the body.

Now moving down to the area around the pubic bone and the lower belly. Being aware of this area and then moving to the side of your body, the back of your body; the lower back, and the other side of your body. Now move your awareness to your lower arm and then the other lower arm, around the wrists, into the palms, over the back of your hands and along each of the fingers of both hands. Now down to the pelvis and then out to one of the hips, around to the back of the body and then to the other hip.

Move down to your thigh. Take your awareness down the front of your thigh, around to the side, the back of your leg and then to your inner thigh. Repeat this for the other leg. Keep bringing your mind back every time it wanders.

Move your awareness down to one of your knees. Take your mind around the front of the knee, then the side of the knee and around to the back and then the other side. Repeat this process for the other knee.

Now move down to your lower leg, starting at the front, moving to one side, around to the back and then to the other side. Then repeat this process for the other lower leg. Moving down to your ankle. Working around the front, the side, the back and other side of the ankle and then going on to the other ankle.

Moving your awareness to the top of one of your feet. Then to the heel and the sole of the foot, and moving across each of your toes in turn, starting with the big toe. Now repeat this on the other foot.

Finally take your awareness back to your crown and quickly sweep your awareness down through your whole body all the way down to your toes. Make a mental note of each area of your body in turn but be relaxed and present. You are just noticing how your body feels in this moment. You may like to repeat this sweep through the body several times. Just be natural and allow the mind to flow with the breath.

Bring your mind back to your hara and place it deep into this area. Notice the rise and fall of the belly with each breath.

Now extend your awareness out into the room that you are in. Take a few slightly deeper breaths than normal and feeling your connection to the earth. Firstly, moving your hands, your feet and then in your own time opening your eyes ready to resume your normal daily activities.

There are many different approaches to the Body Scan, and all are equally valid. Feel free to try a different approach if the Japanese method is not to your liking. An interesting variation on the Body Scan meditation for Reiki practitioners is to take your mind around the energy channels or meridian system within the body. Whilst this does mean that you are following wherever the meridian leads rather than from the top of the head down to the feet as in a traditional Japanese approach to the Body Scan, in this form the meditation does become a powerful healing mechanism. You would need to familiarise yourself with the body's meridian system first to be able to practice the meditation. It is quite complex for those who have not studied it before, but well worth the effort.

During the Body Scan meditation as with the others in this book, you probably noticed again how your mind wandered all over the place, filling with random thoughts and idle speculations about the future or memories of the past. In our attempts to experience life directly we should be aware of not trying to prevent these thoughts from arising or from attempting to force them out of our minds. Thoughts are as much an aspect of our lives as any other and need to be accepted into the totality of our experience along with everything else. We should, however, avoid identifying with them too closely.

Our ability to see the world (or in this case, our own bodies) from the perspective of unmediated direct awareness, clearly demonstrates that we are not our thoughts. Thoughts happen to us, like the weather. They are mental events, no more than scratches on the acetate projecting onto the cinema screen of our mind. Normally when we have a thought, we tend to believe what it's telling us. We buy into it and identify with it and we look at the world from its perspective. If we are sat meditating and the thought arises "I don't have time for this," we tend to believe it and the body then responds accordingly. We might start to feel a little tension building up in the neck area as we follow the thought train into "I need to get that report done or I will never meet the deadline." Perhaps our breathing has also started to respond to the thoughts, and it has lost the relaxed and restful quality that it had a few moments ago. Before we know it, we've given up on our meditation and are sat at our desk working. We can see from this remarkably familiar experience of being human that thoughts constantly influence our feelings and the sensations that we experience in our bodies. It is also true that thoughts are in turn influenced by the feelings and sensations experienced in our bodies. There is a symbiotic relationship between the two.

When examining our own discomforts, aches or pains we should try to keep in mind that the thoughts that we have about our experiences are not us. These mental events are separate from us and they are not necessarily true. Remember that thoughts are not facts, even the ones that say they are. Mindfulness allows us to notice our thoughts without buying into them and believing everything they have to say. In the same way, we can also step back and detach from our emotions. As we saw in Chapter 2, we are no more our emotions than we are our thoughts. We can gain a great deal of freedom and clarity of mind by learning to detach from our emotions and bring the laser focus of our awareness to them.

I am sure that when Mikao Usui put together the Reiki Precepts it was no accident that he focused very directly on the arising of such negative emotional states as worry and anger which produce such immense amounts of stress and suffering in people's lives and so contribute to profound states of physical and mental ill health around the world. Any good spiritual discipline must surely address these terrible and debilitating mind-states that prevent us from experiencing the true beauty of life and all that we are capable of experiencing.

In our mindfulness practice, we are neutral observers of these emotional events. We can see with awareness how our thoughts have generated negative mind-states such as worry and anger and how in turn they generate new thoughts. When we are angry, we tend to point a finger at whoever or whatever we are angry at and blame them for the way we are feeling. To gain freedom from these emotions we must first learn to take full responsibility for their arising. No one and nothing outside of us can ever generate any kind of emotion within us, though they may trigger within us an experience of a particular emotional response. Just as we saw in relation to our meditation practice earlier on, when we sit, we are profoundly alone in that endeavor. The wall or the back of the chair is not responsible if our physical posture collapses. We shouldn't be relying on the wall or the chair to support us in the first place. The music is not responsible if our focus drifts off into daydream. We shouldn't be relying on the music to get us into a relaxed state in the first place. Other people and circumstances are not responsible if our emotions become destabilised. We shouldn't be giving them power over our emotional stability in the first place.

To explore this, we can resort to a practice called RAIN.[26] RAIN is an acronym for Recognising, Allowing, Investigating and Nurturing (or Non-identification[27]). RAIN is a process designed to cultivate acceptance and ownership of our inner processes.

Recognising

Whenever we have a difficult emotion such as anger or worry arising during our meditation practice, we can turn our attention towards it and acknowledge its presence. We could speak to it and say, "Hello worry." Do not try to avoid the emotion. This will result in a contraction of our awareness as avoidance inadvertently feeds the negative emotions and strengthens them.

Allowing

In this stage we need to be fully open to the experience of the emotion and welcome it in. We need to fully own how it feels. If there is resistance at this stage, we should note it and also allow it into our awareness. In this approach we are embracing the totality of our internal weather systems. Suppression on the other hand kills off any potential there may have been for the arising of insight. Allowing is very much a "being" mode activity whereas suppression is a "doing" mode activity.

Investigate

This is where many people can get led astray and in seeing the label "Investigate" fire up their analytical thinking processes and start to forensically dismantle what is going on in an effort to identify the causes of their emotional state. This is not how we should be approaching this. Instead of thinking about what is happening emotionally, try experiencing what is happening. It's a bit like the exercise we did previously of thinking about our hand and then experiencing what a hand feels like from the inside. Try listening to the body and locating where the emotion is having an effect. What does that feel like? What does it need to start healing?

Nurturing

Once you have gained a feeling for what is needed to heal, you can consciously draw on that deep sense of compassion and wisdom that comes from your true self and embrace your vulnerabilities. You might like to consciously breathe love and kindness into the areas of your body where the emotion is having an effect. Saturate each in and out breath with the quality of love. Surround yourself with soft luminous light. Befriend yourself. Perhaps see a good friend or a parent holding you with love.

Once we have softened the emotion through our nurturing activity, we might find that it simply melts away. This is where we can often spontaneously experience the state of emptiness or non-identification. However, we should be aware that when we look at the emotion again it might return just as strongly as before. When this happens, we need to repeat our practice and do so again and again until we start to strongly connect with the reality that these mental dramas are not us and they are not permanent. They are, like our thoughts, simply internal weather patterns cast against the infinite clarity of our own pure state of being.

The mind's relationship to our pain and suffering is complex. By bringing mindfulness to bear on this relationship, we can begin the process of claiming our freedom from suffering. As practitioners of Reiki, this should be our first priority.

Chapter 7

The Heart of Reiki

It always surprises me just how little practices that develop the quality of love, kindness and gratitude, etc., are focused on in the Reiki literature. Given that many people experience Reiki as a manifestation of love, it seems to me that this quality is central to the practice. It is, in fact, one of its defining principles and expressed in the Reiki Precepts themselves: "Be kind to yourself and others… Be mindful about this in your heart/mind." Without this quality, pretty much everything else in the Reiki system becomes null and void. Of course, vague nods are made in the direction of developing such qualities as love and kindness and compassion by various writers and commentators, but not in any substantive way. No methods are given and it's as if there is an expectation that we can just be nice to each other and that's enough, or that a deeper manifestation of love will spontaneously arise. We *should* be nice to each other of course, but if we are to plumb the depths of what the Reiki system has to offer as a spiritual practice, it is not enough. Not even close to being enough.

One of the primary tools and focus points for the committed practitioner of Reiki is the heart. This is the universal center of love; the seat of the divine descended to the depths of the human heart and manifesting in a way that is accessible and understandable to us as human beings. If you ask a Sufi where it is that he is looking for God, he will tell you: in his own heart. If we look back at the Reiki symbols, we find the *bindu* point, the termination of Symbol 1 as it winds through the *chakra* system, at the heart. This is the location of *Dai Ko Myo* – the Absolute; the state of complete perfection and oneness with the universe; our own Buddha Nature – the great bright light, identified with Dainichi *Nyorai*: The Sun or Cosmic Buddha. Many people describe the energy of Reiki as love. So, it makes sense that the heart is a primary focus for development for all practitioners of the discipline of Reiki. If we don't develop the heart, how can we truly express this profound quality of love that is at the heart of our discipline?

For those familiar with the *chakra* system, you will know that the name for the Heart chakra is *Anahata* (the location of the middle elixir field of the *hara* system; that swirling, pulsating ball of energy which is a gathering place of both *yin* and *yang*). As was mentioned earlier in the chapter on the Reiki symbols, *Anahata* is also another name for the *mantra* or seed syllable/ *bija*, *Om*. *Om* is the unstruck sound. *Om* generates itself and requires only itself. From the vibration of *Om* everything in the universe emerges: sound, or the vibration that we perceive as sound, creates form (according to the *Upanishads*; the ancient Hindu texts: "In the beginning was the sound, and the sound was Om"[1]). *Om* is, according to the *Upanishads*, another name for Brahman or God. More correctly it is the sacred syllable that represents God,[2] it is an expression of the Absolute.

If we work with the *mantra Om*, we find that there are four parts to it. *Om*, when verbalised, is sounded as *Aum*. The "A" starting at the back of the throat, the "U" resonating on the upper palate and the "M" at the lips. These three parts to the *mantra*, leading us through the three states of our ordinary consciousness, finally give way to the fourth part: the silence that pervades everything; the *anusvara* (after-sound). This silence is the transcendent state of consciousness; the Absolute. It is the ultimate expression of *Om*. It is described in the *Maitrayaniya Upanishad* as "tranquil, soundless, fearless, sorrowless, blissful, satisfied, steadfast, immovable, immortal, unshaken, enduring."[3]

As we have seen in relation to the Reiki symbols, the Absolute is identified with Dainichi *Nyorai* (*Dai Ko Myo*) and that *Om* is also identified with Dainichi through the *Dharmakaya* (as we saw in relation to Symbol 2). We can see therefore that there is a direct equivalence between *Om* and *Dai Ko Myo* as personified in Dainichi *Nyorai* and thus there is a direct relationship between the divine principle (Dainichi *Nyorai*) and the heart (*Anahata*). Further, we see that Symbol 2 has a relationship with Symbol 3 through *Om's* relationship to the *Hon* of *Hon Sha Ze Sho Nen*. *Hon* references the true source of *Sha,* which is me or I, myself. So, by unpacking *Hon Sha Ze Sho Nen* and *Sei Hei Ki* we can hope to one day realise our *Dai Ko Myo* (*Om*) at the *bindu* point of *Choku Rei.*

The heart then is the location within the human energy matrix where we need to place our focus or make a journey towards within our practice of Reiki if we are to develop the transcendental state of oneness with the universal mind: which is the ultimate goal of the Reiki system. As we all know, the fundamental quality associated with the heart is love (it is no coincidence that when we wind the *Choku Rei* through our *chakra* system, we find its termination point; the *bindu,* at the heart).

In placing Dainichi at the center of our heart, we are in a sense confronting his radiance all of the time. However, in confronting it, or observing it, we are limited by our dualistic orientation and thus cannot be at the center ourselves. Our difficulty is that there is an "I" which is standing apart from the Absolute. We experience the Absolute as something that is outside of ourselves. Because we are identifying with our physical body so closely, everything that is not us is separate from us and thus, as Vessantara has said "is the dark well-spring of all suffering."[4]

According to Vessantara there is a way to resolve this problem, a practice that can help us to realise our true nature as one with the Absolute, and that is through the development of loving kindness, which links us straight back into the importance of the Reiki Precepts as a central and foundational aspect of the Reiki system:

> *It involves giving up all attempts at power and control and relating to the world through loving-kindness. It is this turnabout*

> *in our attitude which is required by the first precept taken by all Buddhists. It is usually expressed in negative terms as undertaking not to harm living beings. However, if we plumb its significance to the depths, we see that there is far more involved than not blacking eyes or swatting flies. It involves giving up the central place we give to our egotistical interests and concerns, not using even the subtlest force or manipulation to obtain what we want but relating to the world and other people with a co-operative spirit, from a basis of loving-kindness.* (Vessantara, 1998)[5]

The development of loving kindness, or *metta* is embodied within the teachings of the Buddha in the *Karaniya Metta Sutta.*[6] In this text, the Buddha enjoins us to develop universal love for all beings without exception. The practice of *metta* is common to all schools of Buddhism but is elevated to a much greater degree within the Mahayana schools and often conflated with the quality of compassion, which together with wisdom is considered to be the path to enlightenment.[7]

The Dhammapada[8] says "Hatred cannot coexist with love and kindness. It dissipates when supplanted with thoughts of love and compassion." The practice of loving-kindness or *metta* is the ultimate method for expressing selfless love and generosity towards ourselves and others and ridding ourselves of the negative emotions that cause us and others to suffer so much. They melt away in the light of it as they cannot exist beside it.

The need for love is a biological necessity. As we grow, we need to be touched, we need care, we need to be hugged and to be acknowledged by others. When we are deprived of these things, we are deprived of the chance to live a healthy life. This is not only on an emotional and psychological level, but also on a physical level. The word *metta* is derived from another word: *mitta,* which means "friend." It also means "sun."[9] And just as we rely on the sun's warmth to survive, we also rely on the love and friendship of others for our health and wellbeing.

The Buddha described how we need to practice if we are to experience the quality of *metta* in our own lives. Firstly, we generate the quality of loving-kindness for ourselves and then we generate it for others. We are not, however, talking about ordinary love in our *metta* practice. It's a type of love that we not only feel throughout our whole being, but also has no ulterior motive. It doesn't change when the person to whom we are feeling this love changes. When the person that we are feeling loving-kindness for does something bad, our *metta* should not give way to disappointment or anger or hatred. If it does, it was never *metta* in the first place. *Metta* arises from a pure heart, and it is the purification of the heart that we are striving to realise in our practice of Reiki.

Sharon Salzberg had this to say about *metta*:

> *the spirit of Metta is unconditional: open and unobstructed. Like water poured from one vessel to another, metta flows freely, taking the shape of each situation without changing its essence. A friend may disappoint us; she may not meet our expectations, but we do not stop being a friend to her. We may in fact disappoint ourselves, may not meet our own expectations, but we do not cease to be a friend to ourselves.* (Salzberg, 1995)[10]

The kind of love that we are describing here has qualities that distinguish it from our usual experiences of love, which are often mixed with desires or attachments. *Metta* does not seek self-benefit or something in return. It's not an exchange: "I will love you if you act the way that I want you to act," or "I will love you if you love me."

In the *Metta Sutta*, the Buddha gave an example of the quality of loving kindness that is to be aspired to. A mother will watch to see if her child is hungry and provide food even before the child asks for food. If the child is in danger, she will risk her own life. So, the Buddha asked us to love all beings as a mother would love her only child. This is, of course, a very difficult thing to do. One of my students in Egypt during a class discussion about the practice of *metta* could not at all conceive of even the possibility of feeling the sort of love and kindness towards another person that she naturally feels for her own children. It is necessary, however, if we are to develop genuine *metta*. *Metta* is not discriminatory. There are no levels to *metta* where one is more deserving than another, or that a "lesser" quality of love is more appropriate for one person as opposed to another. We cannot dissolve the barrier between "self" and "other" or become a true expression of *Dai Ko Myo* at the center of the *Choku Rei*, which is a primary goal of the Reiki system, whilst we believe that one person is deserving of a lot of love, and another of much less love (or none). This simply perpetuates the dualistic illusion that we are all separate and looking out only for ourselves. But if we truly wish to see through this illusion then, perhaps, we should look at some characteristics of *metta* which might help us.

Many people seem to regard the generation of *metta* as being something ephemeral, lacking in real substance; a sort of floaty feeling of loveliness for others, but as we have seen, this is not *metta*. *Metta* is very much a feet-on-the-ground hard core expression of real deep love. When you feel *metta* towards someone, you don't want them to just be happy, you want them to be deeply happy, backed up by an ardent desire for their welfare, their growth and progress, just as a mother does for her only child. *Metta* is without limit and is completely unconditioned by our own state of being, our personal desires or our emotional state. There should be a sort of explosive intensity in our practice of *metta*.

If we think of negative emotions such as anger, hatred, fear, jealousy and despair, we know from our own experience just how much energy these emotions contain. In the *Itivuttaka*, which is a collection of sayings from the Buddha in the Pali

Canon, the Buddha says of *metta*: "it burns and shines and blazes forth."[11] There is clearly an intensity or incandescence of passion being suggested here of the sort that is normally characteristic of our negative emotions. *Metta* then is not some wishy-washy "feeling lovely" about other people sort of quality (though this, of course, isn't a bad place to start, as long as we realise that we are still at the start of our journey). The practice of the development of *metta* is a hard-core commitment to the cultivation of a transcendent quality.

> *Metta brings together the contrasting emotional reactions of dynamic energy and calm repletion into a single quality of emotion, completely transforming them in the process. Although, when it is fully developed, Metta is a feeling of harmony, both in oneself and with all beings. It also has a fiery, full-bloodied, even ecstatic quality. Ecstasy literally means a sense of standing outside oneself, and this is how Metta can feel: it is marked by such an intensity of positive emotion that, when purely felt, it can carry you outside of yourself. Metta is blissful, ecstatic, a naturally expansive desire to brighten the whole world, the whole universe, and universes beyond that.* (Sangharakshita, 2004)[12]

The purpose of such intensity of practice is to help us gain insight into the true nature of reality, to enable us to gain an appreciation for our own true nature as an expression of the Absolute. *The Metta Sutta* is essentially divided into three parts. Each part has a very distinct focus. The first part of the *Sutta* expresses the need for the generation of loving-kindness through the way that we conduct ourselves. The second part is very much concerned with the development of *metta* as a method to achieve *samadhi* or a higher state of consciousness, which is brought about by an absorption into the feeling of *metta* itself. The third part requires complete commitment to the concept of universal love as expressed through all bodily, mental and verbal activities. When we practice generosity, forgiveness, kindness to others, our practice of *metta* "ripens" the merit that is produced as a consequence of the practice of these "perfections" (*paramitas*).

> *Metta cetovimutti – universal love leading to liberation of mind – signifies the attainment of samadhi, absorption based upon meditation on metta. Since metta liberates the mind from the bondage of hatred and anger, selfishness, greed and delusion, it constitutes a state of liberation. Every time one practices metta, for however short a period, one enjoys a measure of freedom of mind. Measureless freedom of mind, however, is to be expected only when metta is fully developed into samadhi.* (Buddharakkhita, 1995)[13]

So, our practice of *metta* is very much linked to the realisation of the Reiki Precepts, with the use of the symbols as meditative devices to aid us in the task of developing true *metta* or being absorbed into *metta* as a way to the heart or a realisation of the true nature of reality. Practicing *metta,* or indeed any other aspect of your work with the Reiki system should not be just an intellectual exercise. It requires a full commitment to making it your guiding philosophy through life so that it impregnates every aspect of your daily life: your attitude, your outlook on life and the way that you conduct yourself. It should be at the core of your meditation practice, thus at the core of your engagement with the system of Reiki. The development of *metta* is an activity that requires the mind coming fully to bear on the activity of the mind. We must continually watch our mind and guard it. When we are aware of our mind and can come from a place of love and purity, *metta* is cultivated very intensively.

We have looked at the expression of *metta* towards others in terms of its quality and intensity and that it is a gateway to a realisation of the Absolute; the dissolution of "self" and "other" and all dualistic concepts. We therefore need to consider our relationship to the practice. If we stop looking at the practice from our normal dualistic perspective: "I" feel loving kindness for "you," then we see that there is no "I" to feel *metta* and there is no "you" for me to express *metta* to. There is only *metta*. When we fully embody this experience of deep, powerful loving kindness, we fully embody the state of *metta* and become absorbed into it. We become immovable in our state of singular absorption into this profound state. When an enemy or someone that has harmed us is the subject of our *metta* practice, it can be very difficult to feel profound loving kindness for them. We might be able to dispel our hatred or our dislike and feel forgiveness towards them and be willing to gingerly extend the hand of friendship towards them, but this is not *metta*. *Metta* is completely undisturbed by the nature of the person who we are feeling *metta* for. *Metta* simply is. In fact, *metta* requires no object. The goal of our practice, as already stated, is to simply merge into the quality of *metta* and be still. Nothing and no one should be capable of disturbing the expansive and infinite stillness of profound love that we aspire to embody. While we hang on to the concept that someone or something is capable of disturbing our *metta*, then we are still not yet fully absorbed into the experience of *metta*. *Metta*, like the Buddhist *vajra* is indestructible, diamond-like, pure, and utterly without end or beginning. In this sense then we can truly embody the sort of love that a mother has for her only child. It becomes an indestructible quality. We can think of the sun shining and radiating light through space in this respect. When a planet crosses its path, the sun shines on it and the planet is bathed in light. If there is no planet, the sun still shines. Whether there is something to radiate light to, or whether there is not, is irrelevant, the sun shines anyway. This is how we should aspire to be with our *metta*. We shine anyway. When we do so, there is an infinite expanding flow of *metta* that bathes anyone and anything that comes into its path. So, our practice of *metta* is not so much a state of mind but a movement within our consciousness: a movement of dazzling, brilliant radiance.

Simply being nice to everyone is of course then clearly not our ultimate goal, but this is where we must start, and it is an excellent place to start. It should be kept in mind, however, when we select someone as the object of our *metta* practice, we do not base that selection on the basis of any cause or justification. We are not selecting people that we like or ignoring those that we don't like. It really shouldn't matter who we select. Sangharashita again:

> *When we practice the metta bhavana, our feelings of good will towards beings do not arise on account of anything those beings may have said or done. We simply wish them well. If it were otherwise, metta would be no more than a psychological thing, coming and going in dependence on whom we bring to mind at any one time. As a spiritual quality, metta is not bound by any kind of stipulation or qualification or condition. It is not meted out according to whether beings deserve it or not.* (Sangharashita, 2004)[14]

We should aim to express *metta* regardless of what someone does or does not do. As Sharon Salzberg made clear,[15] when we can simply embody *metta,* regardless of the object of our practice, love becomes the natural state of our own being. We become naturally connected and naturally at peace. Love becomes the reflection of who we are.

An important quality of the practice of cultivating *metta* is that we can use it to support our practice of mindfulness meditation. In doing so it helps the mind to stay open and sweet. It brings a softness to our practice and provides the essential balance that our insight practice needs. In an intensive practice of *metta,* we find that we are radiating loving-kindness all the time in whatever position or situation that we find ourselves in, whether that be sitting, standing, walking or lying down. As we walk along, for instance, we simply radiate *metta* to everyone and anyone that passes us, or we are aware of in our vicinity. As the action of walking requires energy, this helps to keep the arising of *metta* in a sustained and constant state of flow. It is, of course, necessary, whether we are walking or cultivating *metta* in the standing or seated or lying down posture, to bring the quality of loving-kindness to ourselves first. There is a profound psychological reason for this. No one that hates, despises or dislikes themselves, consciously or unconsciously can really feel genuine loving kindness for others. I have one student who is utterly focused almost all the time on helping others to the complete exclusion of herself. This is not a good practice. Whilst she gets the gratitude and thanks of those that she is trying to help (and she is only helping them in a very limited way), this simply feeds into her ego and does nothing to dispel the deep need she has for self-love and appreciation that she routinely denies herself. This sort of focus mitigates against an ability to feel genuine loving-kindness for others as there is always a psychological pay back that must be made in exchange for that love. It is vital that we make ourselves the first subject of our *metta* practice, to melt the need to have recognition and acknowledgement from others in exchange for our practice directed at them.

Before we get to the meditation for this chapter, it is worth taking some time to look at some of the benefits of the practice in relation to our journey with Reiki. After all, Reiki is a healing system, even when we view it as a profound set of spiritual tools rather than as just a simple hands-on energy healing method.

Studies on the health benefits of practicing the *metta* meditation are now quite extensive. A landmark study by Barbara Fredrickson in 2008 showed that practicing the *metta* meditation increased feelings of love, joy, contentment gratitude, hope, amusement and awe. The consequence of the arising of these emotions increased the benefits from a wide range of human resources such as mindfulness, purpose in life and social support. These improvements in personal resources predict and were measured to show increased life satisfaction and reduced depressive symptoms.[16] A study at the Duke University Medical Center in the USA tested an eight-week *metta* programme for people with chronic lower back pain. There were significant improvements in the levels of pain felt and the psychological distress associated with the pain, even after the experiment ended. It was also noted that practicing the *metta* meditation on one day, would lead to lower levels of anger the next day.[17] A 2014 study by Tonelli et al. demonstrated the benefits of the *metta* meditation for those who suffered from chronic migraine.[18] The study showed that not only was the pain associated with the migraine reduced but also that the tension associated with it was alleviated. It has also been shown that practicing the *metta* meditation can slow the aging process.[19] As a consequence of the stress reduction brought about by the regular practice of *metta* meditation, women in a study conducted by Hoge et al. (2013) showed relatively longer telomere length compared to age-matched controls.[20] Telomeres are bits of genetic material that are biological markers of aging. Stress reduces telomere length. So, forget all those anti-aging creams, save yourself some money and practice *metta* meditation instead. Finally, a review by researchers in Germany and the US suggested that practicing the *metta* meditation "may provide potentially useful strategies for targeting a variety of different psychological problems that involve interpersonal processes, such as depression, social anxiety, marital conflict, anger, and coping with the strains of long-term caregiving."[21]

There is, in fact, a huge amount of information and data out there now on the benefits of practicing *metta* meditation. Researchers around the world are finding time and time again, that practicing the *metta* meditation is having a profoundly positive impact on the health and psychological wellbeing of meditators all around the world. The *metta* meditation therefore is not only a tool to be used for our spiritual advancement but also something that we can use to enhance and improve our day-to-day health.

Some would say that there is no evidence that Mikao Usui included the practice of *metta* in his teachings. I would disagree. We have seen very clearly that the *Bodhisattva* Kannon (Avalokiteshvara) has a powerful link to both Symbol 2 and Symbol 3. In Symbol 2, Kannon represents the *Sambhogakaya* of the Three *Kayas*. That is, he represents the blissful state of immeasurable loving-kindness and compassion that we should be aspiring to in our practice when we travel the journey of the Three *Kayas* (*Sei-Hei-Ki* in embodying the Three *Kayas* allows us to move from the *Nirmanakaya* to the *Dharmakaya* with the *Sambhogakaya* [Kannon]as an intermediary). In Symbol 3 (which is linked to Kannon) we see that the syllable *Hon* is a signifier for the whole of *Sei-Hei-Ki*, whilst *Sho* relates to the truth of our heart of compassion and *Nen* is a true wish or blessing coming from the heart. So, we can see that Kannon embodies the sublime state of infinite love and compassion that is symbolised within two of the Reiki symbols. To fully realise the qualities associated with these symbols therefore, as embodied in the form of Kannon, we need to engage with a practice whose focus is on the development of transcendent loving-kindness. Within the Buddhist canon, the *metta* practice is the supreme method for doing precisely that.

As stated in Chapter 1, it does seem that Usui introduced mindfulness to his students at the start of their training, and the *metta* practice is an established and intrinsic part of any good mindfulness practice. I once had a conversation with Reiki Master Ranga Premaratna and during that conversation we talked about the importance and need for basic mindfulness instruction at the start of a student's journey into Reiki. He said that since he was a Buddhist, he always worked on the assumption that this was core to the practice anyway, as Reiki is clearly established on a foundation of mindfulness. Mikao Usui was also a Buddhist and likewise the practice of mindfulness and thus the *metta* practice would have been a given in his system. Students would either come with this practice already firmly embedded (if they were Buddhists) or it was taught if they were not familiar with it. The cultivation of *metta*, implicit and deeply embedded within the practice of mindfulness, is also implicit in every aspect of the Reiki system.

Metta practice is a profound and very important part of the Buddhist canon. It deals with the development of the heart and of the quality of love. This is utterly central to the practice of Reiki, as the primary force and focus within Reiki is also the development of love. It is simply not credible in any sense at all that *metta* is not a deeply interwoven aspect of the Reiki system. Without the development of *metta* there simply is no Reiki, just as there is no Reiki without the foundation of mindfulness. As Jack Kornfield said in his classic *A Path with Heart*:

> *All… spiritual teachings are in vain if we cannot love. Even the most exalted states and the most exceptional spiritual accomplishments are unimportant if we cannot be happy in the most basic and ordinary human ways, if, with our hearts, we cannot touch one another and the life we have been given… so that we can say on whatever day is the end of our life, "Yes, I have lived my path with heart."* (Kornfield, 1994)[22]

So how do we practice the cultivation of *metta*, or loving-kindness? Certainly, we should try to carve out a chunk of time to practice each day. Even if it is for just a few minutes, this is fine. You might like to put a timer on this and set it for two minutes or five minutes or whatever works best for you. Once you have decided how long you will sit for, it's a good idea to be consistent and stick with the practice at the allotted time each day. Commitment to developing the quality of love in your daily life is important, so you should try to build it into your daily routine and practice of Reiki. We have already discussed the various meditation postures, so whatever posture is going to work for you, you should adopt. Then we need to consider who it is that we are going to use as our "target"; someone to whom we can radiate *metta*. Certainly, we should start with ourselves and try to feel genuine love and care. You can repeat some positive statements that will help reinforce your intention of generating *metta* for yourself. You might like to say something like "May I be happy," and "May I be at peace," or "May I be free from suffering." All of these are good affirmative statements to make during your self-directed practice, but don't just say them; really listen to them as you say them. Spend a moment or two trying to really feel what it is like to be genuinely happy or at peace or completely free from suffering. Let that feeling soak into the very fiber of your being. It's important that you consider these phrases as something precious. You don't want to grip onto them too tightly, but nor do you want to pay them no heed and let them slip out of your hand. You should as Sharon Salzberg indicated, cherish them gently, carefully, and pay close attention to them, and try to connect to them.[23] You can do your self-directed *metta* practice while you are giving yourself a Reiki treatment if you wish. The two practices together combine extremely well.

When you have directed loving-kindness towards yourself for a while, you should move on to someone else; someone that you are close to. Someone that it is easy to feel loving-kindness for. This could be your son or daughter, mother or father, husband or wife, and then repeat your practice of trying to feel genuine loving-kindness or *metta* for that person. Bring this person into your field of awareness and allow them to be bathed in *metta*. It is traditionally taught that if the person is still alive, it will help to deepen the level of concentration that you can reach than if you pick someone that has passed on. When you have selected this person, reflect on a likable quality or attribute of this person and see if you can feel happy at their desire for happiness. Repeat the phrases that you used earlier; "May (your friend) be happy," "May (your friend) be at peace," "May (your friend) be free from suffering." Reflect on them and try to feel these qualities as you did before, but now in relation to your friend. If someone else comes into your mind during the practice, you can switch your focus to them for a while.

Next, you should select a neutral person; perhaps someone that you don't know very well. Someone that you don't necessarily feel any strong love for, but neither do you feel any animosity towards them either. It could be someone that you see on the way to work every day or that serves you in a shop. Maybe someone that you see outside walking their dog each morning or that delivers your post. Whoever you choose, go through the same routine that you did for yourself and your friend. Try to keep this person as your neutral subject for some period of time. Try not to switch from one to another too often. As you keep focusing over and over again on this same person, you may find that you end up creating a genuine space in your heart for them.

The next stage of the *metta* meditation practice is to select someone that you find difficult. Someone that has upset you or annoyed you in some way. It is not a good idea to pick someone that you truly can't stand the sight of. You are setting yourself a huge task with this. Whilst of course we do ultimately want to feel *metta* for everyone, including the people that we don't like at all, focusing on them at the beginning of the practice is like walking up a mountain backwards with a blindfold on and your arms tied behind your back. You are definitely going to fall. So be kind to yourself and pick someone for this stage of the meditation that has irritated you just a small amount. The smaller the irritation, the better as then you stand some chance of succeeding with your practice. Again, use your positive phrases for this person too. If you find that at any point anger or irritation arises towards this person, you can try visualising them as a small child trying to do their best to navigate the problems of life, or you can see them in your mind when they are ill and in need of support and help.

We can of course generate *metta* for anyone that we choose, even groups of people. We could for instance decide to focus on all our teachers, all the people that live in our neighborhood or town, all the people that we went to school with, our work colleagues. All those that are suffering. All those that cause suffering. All the animals or birds or fish or insects that inhabit the earth. The list is endless. Eventually we want to be able to expand the scope of our *metta* to include all beings everywhere, so working with groups is a good preparation for that. You might like to try doing the *metta* meditation whilst you are giving someone a Reiki treatment and radiating loving kindness to them. This is a powerful healing mechanism.

Those starting out with the *metta* meditation for the first time might find that the following can at times bring up feelings of irritation or anger. It may feel awkward or you may find it to be something of a mechanical process. If this happens, it is important to be gentle and kind with yourself. Whatever feelings come up, accept them in a spirit of friendliness and kindness towards yourself.

Metta Meditation

Start by assuming your normal meditation posture. Make sure that you are comfortable and that your hands are resting comfortably in your lap. If you wish to support your hands with the aid of a cushion, you may do so. This will help to keep your chest open and expansive.

Now take a few slightly deeper breaths than normal and let your body totally relax. Feel the tension slipping away from your shoulders on each out breath. Then allow your breath to return to its normal state. Now take your awareness around your body and check that your posture is stable and that you have a sense of being grounded. Make sure that your spine is straight and resting comfortably. If you are sat in a chair you might like to sit a little forward of the back of the chair unless you have back problems, then by all means rest against the back of the chair or place a cushion behind your back for support. Make sure that your feet are planted firmly on the floor. If you can't reach the floor, you may place a block or cushion there for your feet to sit on.

Keep letting go of any tension on each exhalation. Make sure that your head is balanced nicely as if you are supporting the sky with the crown of your head. Close your eyes or half close your eyes and let your gaze fall gently a few feet in front of you. There should be a sense of quiet dignity about your posture.

Now bring your attention to your breath, going in and going out. Notice how the process of breathing impacts on your body. Where do you feel it the most? Do you feel it at your nostrils or in your chest? Do you feel the rise and fall of the abdomen? Can you get a sense of your breath in the back of your body? How your breath impacts on your whole physical being? Just stay with the breath for a few moments.

If at any time during this meditation your mind wanders, this is okay. Just acknowledge this and bring your mind back to your breath. Use your breath as an anchor for your awareness every time that it wanders. Then return to the focus of the meditation.

As best you can, let go of any plans or preoccupations that you might have and let your mind be quiet. Bring your focus to yourself in a loving and gentle way. Feel a sense of appreciation for yourself. You may mentally or in your imagination or by visualisation, soak each breath with the quality of love and kindness and see this quality radiating out throughout your whole body; permeating every cell within your body, so that you get a sense of each cell vibrating with love and with health.

You may say to yourself "May I be happy," and then allow that phrase to really sink in. Reflect on it for a few moments. Then you may say to yourself "May I be at peace," and again allow that phrase to sink in and then spend a few moments reflecting upon it. Then you may say to yourself "May I be free from all suffering," and once more allow the phrase to sink in whilst spending a few moments reflecting on what this phrase really means. You may adjust these phrases to suite you.

Stay with this process of radiating loving-kindness and appreciation towards yourself for a few moments. You may if you wish, use the imagery that the Buddha offered and see yourself as a small child being surrounded with love and care.

Now bring to mind someone that you care about. Someone that you find quite easy to love. It could be your mother or father, brother or sister, son or daughter. As you do so, see them surrounded by love and kindness. Get a sense of this quality radiating from your own heart and surrounding this loved person. See them smiling and at ease. You may, if you wish, see them as a small child surrounded by your love and your care. You can again repeat the phrases that we used earlier for ourselves. "May my friend be happy," "May my friend be at peace," "May my friend be free from suffering." And as we say each phrase, again allow each one to really sink in and feel how that resonates within your own heart. Reflect on each phrase for a few moments as you say it. Stay with this person in your mind for a few moments, feeling loving kindness and appreciation for them.

Now let us move on to our neutral person. Recall someone that you do not know particularly well. Perhaps someone that you see in the street every day or on your way to work, or someone in a café that serves you coffee. Try to pick someone that you do not feel any sensual attraction to. It is important that your loving-kindness should be pure and not masked by some other feelings or agenda. Once more, you may see this person as a small child being surrounded by your love and caring and kindness. Again, repeat the phrases; "May this person be happy," "May this person be at peace," "May this person be free from suffering." Once more reflect on the words and try to get a real sense of your desire for their realisation for the benefit of your neutral person. Again, just hold this person in your mind for a few moments.

Let us now move our attention to someone that we find more difficult. This could be someone that has irritated you a little in some way or upset you or said something that you don't like. Do not pick someone that you have strong negative feelings for. Someone that has annoyed you only a little is a better subject for this part of the meditation. Again, you can perhaps see this person as a young child surrounded by your love and affection. Try to get a sense of this person as simply in need of being loved and cared for. Try to genuinely feel for them and radiate metta or loving-kindness towards them. You may like to use the phrases that we have used before. "May this person be happy," "May this person be at peace," "May this person be free from suffering." Just stay focused on this person for a few more moments. If feelings of annoyance or anger come up during this part of the meditation, simply acknowledge them. Try to get a sense of how those emotions feel in the body. Try not to hang on to them or buy into them. Simply be with them. Allow them to be and then pass away. Shining the light of your awareness on these emotions will help to dissolve them.

Even if you find it difficult or impossible to feel genuine loving-kindness for this person at this time, simply continue with the practice as best you can and over time you may notice that your resistance to expressing real affection and loving-kindness for this person begins to melt away.

Now bring your awareness back to your breath. Watch your breath going in and out. Stay with this and really get a sense of where you feel the breath in your body. You may like to soak your breath in love and kindness once more.

Gently bring your awareness back into the room that you are in. Feel the connection with the earth through your feet, or the chair or cushion. Just take a few slightly deeper breaths than normal and then in your own time you can slowly open your eyes. Take a few moments before getting up and resuming your normal everyday activities.

May all beings be happy.

In this meditation, we have covered all the classic categories of the *metta* meditation. When you are familiar with this meditation try to vary it and include groups of people. Whoever is the focus of your meditation, however, it is a good idea to keep them as the focus for some days or weeks. We want to really give ourselves the chance to build up genuine *metta* for a particular person. This is not easy if we are changing the subject of our meditation from day to day.

You may also wish to spend some time doing the *metta* meditation just for yourself for a few weeks before moving on to someone else and focusing on them for a period of time. Experiment with what works best for you.

As you develop your practice you will find that you can practice the *metta* meditation anywhere. Do it while driving your car and radiating *metta* towards all those driving in the opposite direction as they pass you. It's a great way to spend time if you are stuck in a traffic jam or waiting to see a doctor or dentist. You can practice while you wait for a bus or to get served in a supermarket. The more you practice, the more you will feel a genuine sense of loving kindness towards others and the more you will feel a sense of deep calmness and serenity in your daily life which will keep you connected to your heart.

May all beings be happy.

Chapter 8

Form Is Emptiness, Emptiness Is Form

As has been made clear throughout this book, there is a need in the practice of Reiki whilst recognising and celebrating its ability to induce and support healing for others, to turn inwards and look at our own state of suffering. As has also been stated many times, this is its primary function and was the focus of Mikao Usui in developing the system. The whole system of Reiki urges the practitioner to look deeply into the nature of their own suffering with the intention of transforming it into a source of insight to be used as fuel for the development of wisdom and compassion that could ultimately bring benefit and healing to others. This insight is built on the profound realisation (and not just an intellectual acknowledgement) of the impermanence and emptiness of all form. As the Tibetan monk Lama Sangwa said, "Even illness is precious, as it teaches us the transience of all existence... Make use of this body now and recognize the Buddha within."[1] We are all imperfect beings and perhaps it would be wise to view our imperfections as a blessing. Every one of them provides us with rich compost within which we can grow, develop and perfect ourselves which can then empower the process of bringing healing to others.

Our journey with Reiki, therefore, is one that provides us with many opportunities for growth through the application of the various tools within the system: the Precepts that enjoin us to engage with the primary practice of mindfulness meditation, the symbols, our "inner GPS" that provides us with an energetic road map to guide us on our journey and the initiations or attunements/*reiju* that awaken within us our "inner mandala" of subtle energy channels that connect us to the primordial nature of the universe. These initiations are designed to provide us with the fuel necessary to awaken within us the mind's inherent radiant nature. To bring this to conscious fruition, however, we must have a resolute commitment to engaging in our spiritual practice. Concepts such as enlightenment or *samadhi* remain fundamentally abstract and of no value unless we realise them within our own minds and bodies through an engagement with the teachings of the system. You could say that the mind of wisdom that is cultivated as a consequence of working with the system of Reiki, particularly the meditational aspects of it, is the system's ultimate expression of the art of healing, because it is only in this that the delusions that imprison us in the world of *dukkha* can be banished and our True or Buddha Nature, made manifest.

We can say that the twin qualities of compassion and wisdom that arise as a consequence of practicing mindfulness meditation and which are enhanced through its integration with hands-on healing are the natural attributes of the fully awakened mind. The realisation of this blissful state of pure awareness spontaneously gives rise to the desire for the liberation of all beings from the realms of suffering. When we practice Reiki, we can be very aware of the transformative nature of the practice, which is to say the transformative nature of the energy that we are working with. When we contemplate the symbols or the specific archetypal deities they represent and so embody those qualities within ourselves, we are tapping into our own innate human potential to overcome our self-limiting concepts and perceptions. "Resting in the natural radiance of our own Buddha mind, all attachment and subtle clinging dissolves in the nature of self-manifesting light"[2] (Baker, 1997). Thus, the realisation of our *metta* practice as discussed in the last chapter is spontaneously achieved: we become *metta* (the essence or principal condition of the Universal Energy Field) and radiate this quality unconditionally for the salvation of all beings.

In his book *Reiki Transmission of Light Vol 1*, Robert Fueston noted in relation to the Reiki attunements/*reiju* that the process activates or energises a pre-existing channel within the body in the same way that electricity might course through already installed wiring once the switch is thrown.[3] This is, however, only a part of what is happening. As we saw in Chapter 4, the attunement/*reiju* process essentially provides a catalyst for the practitioner to connect to their own True Nature and to experience the bliss of merging into the state of Oneness, or the Absolute. Fueston goes on to note how one Reiki teacher described the system of Reiki as just "lazy person's Qigong" and that later a Qigong instructor along with some of his students at a martial arts school commented that it felt as if their Qigong practice had immediately advanced by several years following the Reiki initiation.[4] This is an interesting perspective and there may indeed be some truth in the comment that Reiki is just "lazy person's Qigong" with the ability to advance a student extremely rapidly. We do need to take that with a pinch of salt, however. Reiki isn't just Qigong. It calls on practices embedded deep within the heart of esoteric Buddhism as well as from esoteric Buddhist Qigong. It's very well known that Mikao Usui was himself a Qigong master (though what his precise training and practice was is currently unknown). It's also known that he drew heavily on his understanding of this practice in his development of the Reiki system, though we may never know precisely what he used or what influenced him in any real depth. Mrs Takata, the woman responsible for bringing Reiki to the West in the 1930s, clearly had some knowledge of this and referenced various aspects of the system of Traditional Chinese Medicine (TCM), of which Qigong is an integral part, during her Reiki classes. She almost certainly gained this knowledge from her teacher, Chujiro Hayashi, who was a student of Mikao Usui's.[5] There is no doubt that Reiki owes a great deal to TCM and various branches or schools of Qigong and it is possible that Usui learnt much during his widely reported visit to China.[6]

It's interesting to note that within esoteric Buddhist Qigong there exists the use of the mantra *Om Ah Hum* which we saw in Chapter 3 as having a direct relationship to the Reiki symbols. In Buddhist Qigong the mantra is used in practices such as the "Nine Segment Buddhist Breathing" which is a method for helping the mind to focus on the breath, eliminate all other thoughts and bring the mind of the practitioner into an awareness of and a merging with the "great luminosity of the Cosmos" (Liang & Wu, 1997).[7] As can be clearly seen, it is an aid in the practice of mindfulness meditation. The repetition of the mantra is tied to visualisations linked to the crown *chakra* (the *baihui* point in Qigong), the throat *chakra* (the *tiantu* point in Qigong) and the Heart chakra (the *shanzhong* point in Qigong) and activates the same channels that run along and parallel to the spine that Robert Fueston highlighted as being activated by the Reiki attunement/ *reiju* process. Visualisations as well as self and front generating practices of the *Bodhisattva* Avalokiteshvara, related to so many aspects of the Reiki symbols, also occur within different parts of the Buddhist Qigong cannon.

The activation of the same energy channels that run along the spine also happens as a consequence of engaging in the practice of Deity Yoga. As discussed in Chapter 3, it is probable that Mikao Usui was familiar with and possibly engaged in this practice of self-generating specific deities to realise within himself the inherent qualities of those deities. A requirement for engaging in such practices is the receiving of an empowerment. This esoteric, highly mystical process is the energetic permission to engage with the practice and realise the attributes within oneself of the respective deity. It often involved introducing the student to the mandala or symbol of the particular deity. Without the empowerment, it is believed that the practice would be largely pointless. This is in all respects exactly the same message that has been given since the early days of Reiki in the West in relation to the Reiki symbols, which is that one must be "attuned to them" or they don't work. As we know, the symbols "stand in for" various Buddhist deities, which in turn "stand in for" various attributes of the fully awakened mind.[8]

As a consequence of the attunement/*reiju* process, an experience and awareness of energy that would otherwise take you many years of dedicated practice is gained. The downside of this is that whilst in a Qigong context, wisdom and compassion and a level-headed understanding of the nature of energy and one's place in the "great luminosity of the Cosmos" tends to evolve naturally during the many years of practice, in a Reiki context this rarely happens. Ability is achieved instantaneously through the attunement/*reiju* with no corresponding effort, commitment or learning process. The consequences of this are apparent for all to see and are the main reasons why Reiki often has such a hard time establishing its credibility and why it is often met with derision by practitioners and adherents of much more well established and traditional spiritual teachings.

The goals of Buddhist Qigong and Deity Yoga are the same: to bring about a penetration into the nature of the reality of all phenomena and to merge with the Absolute through a realisation that "form is emptiness, emptiness is form" as is described in the *Heart Sutra*. When we receive a Reiki attunement/*reiju*, we are in a sense initiated into the energy field of the deity associated with the Reiki symbols. If we think of the *Bodhisattva* Avalokiteshvara, for instance, as a consequence of the Reiki attunement/*reiju* we can begin to identify with our own perfected potential as embodied within the wisdom mind of the *Bodhisattva* of Compassion. The overriding characteristic of Avalokiteshvara is, of course, that of love or universal compassion (*metta*/loving kindness). It is an energy that resonates deeply and profoundly within the Heart chakra or the elixir field of the middle *tanden*. *Qi* as it is known within the practice of Qigong comes from the power of love. *Qi* and love are always united, and love is the source of everything. Many people have commented that their perception of the nature of Reiki energy is that it is an emanation of an immense field of love, and that love is its only characteristic (if we look at the three Abrahamic faiths, we see that love is one of God's defining or principal qualities).

When we practice Qigong there is an exchange of energy between the person and the universe. When we practice Deity Yoga, there is an exchange of energy between the person and the universe. As Kenneth Cohen noted in relation to the practice of Qigong,[9] engaging in these practices is a bit like optimising a computer. The practices of both Deity Yoga and Qigong are akin to optimising the human computer or the human mind. This is done by deleting old and unnecessary data (the afflictions of the mind) from the system to allow it to run more efficiently and to raise its potential.

The empowerments that are given in the practice of Deity Yoga, like the attunement/*reiju* that are given in Reiki are, as already noted, a critical element of the practice. No progress can be made within the system without the empowerment.[10] They are designed to awaken within us our potential for Buddhahood, create a strong link to our teacher and to the particular deity that the practice is centered upon. The connection to the deity (in Reiki as a secular practice this is mediated through the symbols) is to bring us to a realisation of our own Buddha Nature which is the *raison d'être* of the practice of Reiki. When we can recognize through this process of self-identification with the divine that the qualities of the deity are also our own qualities, the state of Buddhahood or perfection is actualised. In aiming to realise our Buddha Nature we are in the best position possible for helping others to be free from their own suffering. Such an aim is based on an intense love and compassion which we strive for in our practice of *metta* and so we can take full responsibility for the welfare of all other beings. This is why the primary practice within the system of Reiki is self-healing or self-liberation. Only then will it be possible to manifest the ability to truly lead others to a realisation of their own healing through the application of hands-on healing guided by a mind of wisdom.

We should, however, be careful about this concept of aiming for a specific goal such as enlightenment or the realisation of our Buddha Nature. We live at a time when everything is measured and quantified in terms of attaining or failing to attain goals of one kind or another. We look at data and measure everything. *Have I made progress in this endeavor? Am I there yet? How much further is there to go?* There is a danger of applying this approach to our spiritual practices also. We need to avoid turning our practice into just another thing that we can tick off on our life's "To Do" list or another thing that we can grasp at and form an attachment to. Spiritual practice is not an enlightenment project. If we can let go of this type of thinking and center ourselves on emptiness and simply being, we can discover that there is nothing for us to achieve or not achieve; nothing for us to be for or against; no beginning to our practice and no end to our practice. We could say that even the alleviation of suffering for other beings becomes something that naturally arises out of our practice; from the state of being rather than the state of doing. As we saw earlier, when it comes to working in a healing context with a client, we need to let go of the desire to achieve a particular result and allow the client to make their own journey into healing defined by their own needs and not our judgments.

The skilful means of meditating on the Reiki symbols as a way of accessing inherent qualities of Buddhist deities which symbolise qualities within our own primordial Buddha Nature relies, as we saw in Chapter 3, on our core Reiki practice of mindfulness meditation. Through this practice, the qualities of the symbols and of course the qualities inherent within the Universal Energy Field as it manifests in a coarser form within the subtle energy system of the human being become apparent. By bringing awareness and focus to our experience within the methods and practices of the Reiki cannon (various forms of meditation including meditations on the symbols and hands-on energy applications), we can start to realise, in the first instance, what is known within Qigong as *wuji* (and within Buddhist meditation practices as *calm abiding*). *Wuji* is, in a sense, our goal-less goal. Attainment of *wuji* is to realise the universe within oneself. It is a completely egoless state of non-judgment, non-attachment and utter bliss which is realised through an intense engagement with the practice of *samatha* meditation. This is a practice that is centered in the body. We must always return to our body as this is our reality, our home, our pivot and anchor that has a deep relationship with the elemental forces of the universe. So, we bring our mind to bear on the qualities and material substance of the body as well as the movement of subtle energy through such practices as focusing on the breath or moving around the body in a body scan or reflecting on the nature of our emotions. We can internalise the symbols and apply our hands to the physical self in an effort to transform the emotional and subtle energies of the body and our relationship to them. As Rob Preece noted in *The Psychology of Buddhist Tantra*, if we don't stay in relationship with our body and we attempt to transcend both our body and our feelings, we are likely to end up deceiving ourselves into believing that we have dealt with our problems when all we have done is disassociate from them.[11] We are all aware of emotions such as anger, grief, love or sadness that can be responsible for powerful consequences for our physical bodies, but we rarely view these emotions as simply subtle energy patterns with certain characteristics. These energetic states as manifestations of our subtle energy body require our attention just as much as our physical bodies. Contemplation and reflection on the Reiki Precepts is the way forward in this respect.

As we begin to reflect on our physical being and the nature of our physical reality, we can begin to see that the world around us and our own physical being are not independent of the subtle energy body or of consciousness and that these different aspects of our being come together to form the whole that we call "me." One cannot exist without the others. To dispel the illusion that they are somehow separate things and not related to each other, we need to "open up" our awareness. In a sense, we need to expand our inclusive perspective during meditation which can lead us to a clear seeing of how things really are. This approach to clear seeing or the opening out of the wisdom mind is called *hannya* in Japanese (*prajna* in Sanskrit).

If we look at this in a purely Qigong context, the meditation practice known in China as *Zuo Chan* (*Chan* is known as Zen in Japan) is focused on the cultivation and build-up of *Qi* within the lower *tanden*. This energy is then raised through the Thrusting Vessel (along the spinal cord) to bring about a nourishing and strengthening of the physical body and to mix with and fortify consciousness or *shen*.[12] This then leads to a higher or more rarefied state of consciousness and an opening of awareness that then leads to an opening at the Third Eye *chakra*, leading to a full awakening and a profound realisation of being one with the Universal Energy Field.[13] The extraordinary abilities that are conferred from a purification of the subtle energy body can help us transcend many of our human limitations.

We could say that in realising how different aspects of our being are deeply interconnected and interdependent and how one feeds into and strengthens another, we are once more brought back to the practice of the Three *Kayas* that we looked at in Chapter 3 in relation to the Reiki symbols. Our physical body has very much a relationship to the *Nirmanakaya* which like the body of the physical Buddha, is prone to sickness and ill health but is also the vehicle through which we make our journey through life and in which we sit to meditate. Our subtle energetic body has a relationship with the *Sambhogakaya* which can be blocked and unbalanced but has the potential to lead us to a state of harmony and perfect balance and a state of bliss.

Finally, our consciousness which can be prone to confusion, worry and wandering off into flights of fancy has a relationship with the *Dharmakaya* and so has the potential to lead us to a state of immense clarity and profound insight and wisdom.

An outcome of the process of applying *samatha*-powered mindfulness in our everyday experience of the body, the emotions and the mind and in our Reiki practice generally, is that we start to understand and experience the underlying subtle energy that pervades every aspect of our being. In a sense we could say that all levels of being are simply different qualities or vibrations of consciousness which we can perceive in terms of various qualities or vibrations of subtle energy. In realising this, however, we still need to acknowledge that standing behind and deeply embedded within our experience is the notion that there is an independent "I." This "I" is constantly declaring "Here I am, this is me thinking." But when we contemplate this and bring our awareness to the notion that there is such a thing as an independent "I," we can perhaps start to see that this is nothing more than a label for a collection of different aspects or vibrational qualities that when brought together seem to constitute this thing called "me2 or "I." Neuroscientists will tell you that there is in fact no trace of a "self" in the physical brain. As Christopher Germer noted in his book *The Mindful Path to Self-Compassion*,[14] the brain is buzzing with activity all of the time but how and where consciousness arises out of all this activity is unknown. Wolf Singer of the Max Planck Institute in Germany called the brain "an orchestra without a conductor." When we examine the idea of "self" we can only find brief moments of experience that come and go. There doesn't seem to be a "self" there, just thoughts, feelings, sensations, ideas, impressions. Even the awareness of consciousness itself is transitory. Sometimes we are aware, and sometimes not. The "self" seems to be simply a collection of experiences, both mental and physical, that coalesce around an experience of awareness of consciousness. In Buddhism these various aspects are called *skandhas*.[15] Our practice of Reiki through an engagement with mindfulness meditation and self-healing through the application of our hands to our own bodies is designed to ultimately lead us to the realisation that there is in fact no independent "self." When we can let go of our notions of "self" then healing in its broadest sense will follow. Rigidity around the idea of self will result in diminished wellbeing. Life is constantly changing and so are we. When we look at the *skandhas*, these various aspects of our being, we see can see that they are not fixed independent things but are themselves composed of different elements that are in a constant state of flux that come together to form an apparently independent quality of human existence. If we take the primary aspect of our existence which is the physical material body, we can see that it is composed of solid hard parts, fluid parts, parts that have warmth or heat and parts that move or are fixed within the movement of other parts. None of these parts exist independent of the others, just as the human being or the "I" is not independent of the accumulation of the different elements of our being. We mustn't fall into the trap of thinking that these *skandhas* are qualities or things that we possess, however, because there is in fact no self to possess them. The notion of "self" or the ego arises as a by-product out of the interrelationship of the various *skandhas*, the various elements. When we search deeply for the independent "I" behind the *skandhas* we find that there is nobody there. The Dalai Lama once described this very well when he used the analogy of a car. We can see a car as being one discrete object but on another level, as non-existent and independent of the bits and pieces that go together to make a car (wheels, engine, axle etc.).[16] If we were to take the car apart to search for the inner essence of "car-ness" we would simply have a big pile of bits and pieces on the garage floor, none of which would hold or contain this elusive essence or spirit of "car-ness." We could take the parts apart, reduce them to their base materials but still find nothing that contains this quality or essence of "car-ness." It's just not there. The human being is like this; simply the coming together of various attributes that constitute "I." Embracing the reality of our nonexistence, as fixed and immutable beings we can find our way to freedom from suffering.

In what is widely regarded as one of the world's greatest philosophical texts called *The Fundamental Treatise on the Middle Way Called 'Wisdom,'* the teacher Nagarjuna stated that if we were to search for the Buddha, we would not find him within the complex of physical, mental and emotional attributes that we would recognize as the Buddha. But the Buddha is not to be found anywhere else other than within that same complex of physical, mental and emotional attributes that we would recognize as the Buddha. These attributes (or aggregates) are not in him and he is not in them. So, the question must arise: what Buddha is there?[17]

As we contemplate this and apply the same principles to everything in existence, we can begin to see that everything without exception is empty of independent existence. Everything arises or comes into existence only on the basis of its dependence on the arising or coming into existence of other things. Our realisation of this state of emptiness or *shunyata*[18] is our realisation of *wuji*. This emptiness or *wuji* is simply the play of energy that gives rise to all forms. When we begin our journey of realisation through a development of the mind of wisdom, which operates not on the level of intellect but as a deeply felt experience, then healing and liberation from suffering must naturally follow. We can see then that in a sense our healing journey with Reiki is one towards the realisation that as we engage in the healing process there really is no independent "I" to heal.

So, if there is no "I," who is sitting here reading this book? Who is this writing this book? And who is it that gives and receives a Reiki treatment? We could take the view that like the Kabbalist Kalman in Rabbi Lawrence Kushner's *Kabbalah: A Love Story* that there is only God and that we are just aspects of this divine presence:

> *"In this model, God is… a big circle." He drew another big circle on the place mat, but this time he drew the little circle inside the bigger one. "The little circle, here, still represents you, but see, it is within the big circle of God. You would call this mystical monism. It's all one and it's all God. God is simply all there is. And therefore, the separateness of anyone or anything is illusory because everything is a manifestation of God. God is the ocean, and we are the waves."* (Kushner, 2006)[19]

What we have here is a description of how duality and oneness are co-existent. There are no waves without the ocean, but the ocean is also defined in part by the waves that play across its surface. We can say that there is no "I" whilst asserting with just as much conviction that here "I" am and being right on both counts. We can say therefore that there are two ways in which we can view the concept of "self." The first is that there is a living breathing being, the one that we are very familiar with who is reading this book, that has ambitions, goes to work, is a mother, father, brother, sister, son, daughter, office worker, taxi driver, watches TV, engages in spiritual practices, grows old and eventually dies. This is the self that sits and meditates and if this self did not exist, there would be no point in meditating or practicing any kind of spiritual method at all as there would be no self to benefit from it. When we contemplate our body or our mind, we discover that we are not our body and that we are not our feelings or thoughts and nor are we our memories. The search for an independent "I" separate from all personality characteristics continues and we find that in the end there is nothing that we can pin down as being the thing that owns the body, the mind, the thoughts and emotions. And so, this notion of self gives way to a second version of the concept of self.

This version or different understanding of self we can see from our previous analysis is completely devoid of inherent independent existence and that the "I" that we experience is dependent on the coming together of various components which are themselves likewise dependent on the coming together of other attributes such as our thoughts, predispositions and the labels that we give ourselves (names and definitions such as "intelligent," "carefree," "disorganized," "eccentric," etc.) and various other identifying factors. Everything arises as a consequence of certain energetic attributes of the Universal Energy Field coming together for a time before they once more pass into the void from which they came. This is what happens when we die. Sometimes our identification with "I" is quite nebulous. We might remember a time when we won an award or achieved something great. In circumstances such as these, we have a concept of the self but we are not relating this to the body or the mind but some overarching concept that perhaps embraces these things but is inclusive of much more than just these aspects of our being. The self in this instance is more than the sum of its parts. But where is this self? Again, we cannot find it.

When the Buddha was asked quite directly if there was such a thing as the self, he refused to answer. When he was asked why, he refused to answer that question also and said that to waste time trying to figure out if there is or isn't a self is simply to engage in two extreme forms of wrong view that makes spiritual practice and progress impossible. In answering the question of whether there is a self or no-self, whatever the answer, suffering would inevitably follow. Whether we identify as a separate being and cling to the idea of an independent and separate existence or whether we identify as non-self and cling to the idea of expansively merging with the ocean of oneness, there is still the problem of clinging.

Much more important is to follow the Four Noble Truths and deal with our predispositions towards attachment to anything and everything, including clinging to the concepts of self or non-self. Once we have realised a state of freedom from suffering, who really cares if there is a self or not? The discovery of emptiness and non-self can lead to a profound sense of liberation and a lightness to our way of being as we rest easily into a relationship with all of existence. The harder we cling to our identity as separate beings, the more our suffering condenses into more solid forms in our life. When we sit to meditate or when we apply our hands in a self-healing session it's important to stay level-headed and centered in our practice. We should not use this idea of no-self to just bypass life's problems by asserting that it is all an illusion anyway. This is to miss the true meaning of what is meant by emptiness and no-self and is an abdication of personal responsibility to oneself and others.

One of the issues here is the process of thinking. Our practice of meditation along with a willingness to confront ourselves and wake up to the true nature of reality can help us to untangle all of this. When we meditate, we can see clearly that it is impossible to stop the flow of thoughts. We might slow them up somewhat as we develop in our practice but stopping them altogether will not happen. Here is the crux of the self/no-self dilemma because the holding of either or both concepts relies on the process of thinking which is a deeply flawed means of objectively understanding the nature of reality. As we have seen, thoughts are not facts, they are simply mental events passing across the endless expanse of our awareness. To truly understand the reality of the self/no-self conundrum, we need to step away from this thinking process and simply sit in an open field of awareness. As we sit in this state, we start to realise the co-existent nature of self and non-self and that these are merely concepts arising out of the field of awareness. This will lead to a transformation of our relationship with ourselves and who we are.

A couple of years ago one of my students in Cairo came to me for a Reiki treatment because she had a particularly stressful business trip to New York coming up and felt that Reiki might help to settle her mind and reduce her stress. Early in the treatment, I placed my hand over her Third Eye *chakra* and dropped into an open awareness meditation which became incredibly deep as a consequence of the interaction of my awareness with the flow of energy. As my mind became more and more still, deeper, expansive and lucid, I clearly felt the complete merging of my mind with my student's mind. I remember with great lucidity being aware of the process of this happening whilst it was happening and being awestruck within this experience of two minds merging. My reality in that moment was a liberating, core-deep awareness that there was and always had only ever been one mind: infinite, still and at peace. This endless ocean of emptiness was all that existed for what seemed like a moment but also seemed like an eternity. After this the rest of the treatment was pretty much irrelevant but I went through the motions anyway. After getting up from the treatment bed my student described her mind as being like a glassy pool with not a single ripple of thought on its surface; being utterly clear, expansive and profoundly still. She was in a state of deep and blissful serenity at that moment which was mirrored in her eyes and her whole way of being. Even a Reiki treatment has the potential to lead us to an experience of the Absolute.

The tragedy for most of us, however, is that we take so long to engage in practices that help us to discover who we truly are and to live our actual lives, instead of wasting them in idle speculations about the future and in memories of the past. To use a well-worn but these days largely forgotten phrase from the 1960s: the time is now. The endless ocean of awareness is there for all of us if we are willing to make a little effort.

> *The source of wisdom we discover from the practice of mindfulness, if we allow it, will eventually show us the immense and tragic suffering that stems from unawareness. It will allow us to see, to dwell in, and to treasure that deep peace that lies at the heart of each moment if we have the courage to cultivate awareness, here and now. It will allow us to experience being fully alive – here and now, while we have the chance.* (Williams, et al., 2007)[20]

Open Awareness

When we practice mindfulness meditation, we have two different approaches to it that we can take. We can focus in closely on one thing, becoming utterly absorbed into it to the exclusion of everything else (*samatha*), or we can open out and step back and be mindful of many things in a wider field of awareness. Our awareness can be narrow or broad. We might, for instance, focus in closely on the breath, on the sounds within our environment, the smells coming from the kitchen or the feel of our connection to the chair, the floor or the cushion as we sit to meditate. Or we might rest in allowing all and any of these experiences plus anything else that might impinge on our sensory environment, including thinking and feeling, to arise in our conscious awareness. In this instance our awareness becomes what it always in fact was: boundless.

A narrow focus will naturally result in the exclusion of whatever is not the focus at that moment in time. If we are watching the breath, we are not noticing the sensation of our feet on the floor. If we are focusing on the lapping of the waves on the beach, we are not noticing the warmth of the sun on our back. These things have moved into the background of our awareness. When we take the approach of keeping our awareness more open, however, we are not making any effort to focus on anything in particular. In open awareness we are staying open to anything that arises in our consciousness and giving everything equal weight. We are allowing all things to settle gently on the tip of our consciousness before departing and allowing space for the next experience. This word "allowing" is important. Open awareness isn't something that we make ourselves do. It's something that we ease into. It should feel quite natural.

Having an open awareness is not in opposition to having a more focused awareness. With open awareness there must also be an element of focus. As one thing arises in consciousness, our awareness can switch to a more absorbed or concentrated focus. We can momentarily explore whatever has arisen and then return to our open awareness again. There is a constant shift between one approach and the other. An open awareness approach is often good to build on to the end of something like a Body Scan meditation. After a period of quite intense focus on the experiences of the body, it is quite nice to rest back into open awareness for a while. When we are in this state, we can be conscious of seeing, hearing, tasting, touching, smelling, thinking and feeling as well as having an awareness of being aware. The last of these is very important. When we lose the awareness of being aware, we can once more get lost in the illusion of separation and independent fixed existence as a thought or experience grabs our attention and pulls us back into a stream of connected thought leading us once more down the rabbit hole of duality. Subject and object rear their heads once more, and it is the framework of subject and object that we need to lose. As Jon Kabat-Zinn stated:

> *let's allow the field of awareness to expand infinitely to allow the mind, heart to be boundless, hugely spacious, as big as the sky or space itself, with no beginning and no end, no boundary, no circumference, no periphery. No center. And rather than focusing on anything in particular, just allowing the quality of our awareness to be choiceless. To rest in the non-conceptual knowing*

> *quality of mind itself. Not seeking out anything, not pursuing anything, not rejecting anything and not featuring anything, but like an electromagnetic field so to speak, that would instantly know any perturbation any movement whatsoever that would arise within it.* (Kabat-Zinn, 2019)[21]

This stage in our meditation practice is not easy, however. We can't force it to happen, and we shouldn't be disappointed if it doesn't happen straight away. Try to take a longer view and realise that you actually have the rest of your life to engage with and develop your practice. The following meditation which you can do either on its own or following something like the Body Scan meditation will give you a flavor of the open awareness approach to mindfulness meditation and is a good place to start.

The following meditation is an adaptation of one given in *From Mindfulness to Insight* by Rob Nairn, Choden and Heather Regan-Addis.[22]

For this meditation, it is best to be sat somewhere where you can look out onto a spacious scene. If this is not possible just do the best that you can with whatever environment presents itself to you wherever you are.

Let us once more get established in our meditation posture. Make yourself comfortable and rest your hands comfortably in your lap. If you wish you can place a cushion in your lap to raise your hands to a more comfortable position, keeping your chest open and expansive.

Now take a few slightly deeper breaths than normal and start to feel your body relaxing and letting go of any tension on each out breath. Feel your shoulders relaxing and feel your body giving itself up to gravity. Really feel the weight of your body settling down on to the cushion, the floor or the chair. Gently take your mind around your body and check that your posture is stable and that you have a sense of being grounded. Make sure that your spine is straight and resting into its natural S-shaped curve. If you are sat on a chair you might like to sit a little forward of the back of the chair, unless you have back problems then by all means place a cushion there as support for your back. If you are sitting on a chair, make sure your feet are planted firmly on the floor or place a cushion or meditation block under your feet if you cannot reach the floor.

Check your shoulders. Let go of any tension on each exhalation. Check that your head is balanced. Imagine that you are supporting the sky with the top of your head. There should be a sense of quiet dignity about your posture.

Breathing slightly deeper than normal, bring your awareness to your breath. As you breathe in, imagine that your awareness is expanding and on each out breath, breathe that awareness out into the space in front of you. If you have any health conditions that might be impacted by breathing slightly more deeply than normal, then you should simply breathe normally. Have the sense that you are arousing or bringing to life your awareness on each in breath and then releasing that awareness into the space in front of you on each out breath. Do this for maybe fifteen or twenty consecutive breaths. Don't worry if you lose your focus, or your mind wanders. Just acknowledge this and bring it back to the process and carry on from wherever you were.

Now just gaze gently out into the space in front of you. Stop meditating. Stop doing anything special. Just relax on your chair or your cushion and enjoy the scene in front of you. You are not focusing on anything. Not attaching to anything. If the sky is particularly beautiful or the sound of the birds particularly inspiring, then note it, and let it go. If there is the sound of cars rushing by and its unpleasant, don't try to block it out. Note it and let it go. Notice the space in front of you, and around everything. Be expansive in your awareness and keep bringing your mind back every time it wanders.

Now close your eyes and become aware of your internal space. Notice any thoughts or emotions or perhaps bodily sensations. No need to engage with them. Simply note their presence and let them go. Let your body be still and notice how it is feeling in this moment. Make a mental note of this and let it go. Be aware of the temperature of the body and any places of tension or resistance or aches or pains. Allow softness to seep into these areas. Allow your eyes and brow and face to soften and settle back into this space of expansive inner awareness. There is nothing you need to do right now, just be open and expansively aware of your whole inner environment. Just be in stillness. If your mind gets caught up in thoughts or feelings, then you may open out to the external space once more and repeat the breathing process and rest your awareness on your external environment for a while, before internalising your consciousness once more.

Dissolve whatever separates your internal world from the external world. See these two experiences merging into one experience; just sit with it. No need to do anything. Just gaze out into space, utterly aware and stay like this for as long as you wish.

Bring your attention back to your body and its connection to the earth through the cushion or the chair. Notice your breath and then come back into your center, in this moment. Take one or two breaths, moving as you wish when you are ready and then continuing with the rest of your day.

Chapter 9

Reiki Alchemy

Mindfulness meditation is not something that we should be doing just a couple of times a day or only when we are giving someone a healing session. If we want to work in a genuine way with the Reiki system and explore its potential as a spiritual development practice and not just pay lip-service to this idea as is so often the case, we need to make the effort to integrate our practice of mindfulness meditation into our daily lives as much as we possibly can alongside any energy-based work we might be doing. Certainly, if we choose to work with Reiki as a healing therapy, we should be bringing mindfulness fully into the therapeutic setting. Every part of our healing work should be saturated with awareness. Reiki is not and never was simply an energy healing discipline, of course, as should now be quite apparent. Perhaps this is where we need to pause for thought and reflect on why we practice Reiki in the first place and what we hope to gain from it. What is our ultimate objective? Would it even be appropriate to see hands-on healing as the ultimate expression of the system or the goal of the practice as most clearly do? We are all different and all engage with life in different ways and certainly we express that engagement according to our own inner motivations and predispositions. For some, the practice of Reiki is most certainly an opportunity to bring healing to those in need through the use of universal energy transmitted via the hands. However, it is not the case that this should or must be your objective when working with the system of Reiki.

Over the years, quite a number of my students have come to me with the desire to learn Reiki but with no desire whatsoever to give treatments to others. When they ask the question, there is often a look of quiet guilt on their face. After all, Reiki is an energy-therapy for helping others, right? Isn't that the whole point of it? Who would not want to give Reiki treatments? I always smile and tell them: me! My passion in the system of Reiki is in teaching it to others and empowering them to change their own lives and to take full responsibility for that remarkable alchemical process. I have no real interest in being a Reiki therapist. That said, over the years I have given hundreds of treatments and seen significant changes in many people's lives. Some of these changes are truly miraculous. I do, however, tell all of my students that it is perfectly acceptable to learn Reiki for the sole purpose of engaging with it as a set of tools for their own personal journey of liberation through life and that it is more than okay not to have any intention to give other people Reiki treatments. This is often a huge relief, many of them lighting up at this news. Often these people have been searching for a meaningful spiritual practice for a long time and when they find Reiki, hope that it might be that practice providing them with what they need to bring a sense of peace and harmony and wellbeing into their own lives. Often these people are in dire need of personal healing and personal transformation and it is not acceptable at all to foist on them the notion that to learn Reiki requires a commitment to working on others as an energy healer. It doesn't. Of course, it has to be acknowledged that in the long run, many of these people will almost certainly want to try their powerful healing abilities on someone else, even if just out of curiosity and, of course, this should be encouraged. There are also times when it becomes very clear that because of their own inner healing needs, the last thing some people should be doing is practicing Reiki on others. Not because they can cause any harm, but because their priority needs to be their own urgent healing process. In this instance I actively discourage them from giving other people treatments until they have worked on themselves and brought some balance to their own body/mind complex.

Of course, progress towards that goal cannot be gained without some degree of effort. Dedication and regularity in the practice enables us to better face life's obstacles with courage and confidence as we begin to develop more trust in the process. Staying within the framework of the practice is all down to self-discipline and a daily commitment to do the best that we can. We shouldn't give up because it all seems too hard. We can, after all, check in on our state of being quite easily by tuning into the sensations within our bodies which will give us immediate feedback on the state of our mental and emotional wellbeing at any time. One cautionary note, however; just like placing a pot on the stove, it is never going to boil if we keep taking it off. Consistency and commitment are paramount, and a letting go of any goal or outcome that we may have devised for ourselves. Just be with the process and flow with it.

It can often take a lot of courage to acknowledge the need for personal healing or personal recovery from trauma or physical pain. Given the power of the Reiki system, this process of change and transformation can sometimes be dramatic and may be very traumatic in its speed and depth. Anyone can learn to be a Reiki therapist. It's very easy. On the other hand, it's often not so easy to face oneself and commit to the process of self-transformation or self-healing. Even in this, however, it should be recognized that a commitment to personal transformation is also an expansive commitment to the healing of the world around you. You cannot heal one without the other. If we spend time working on ourselves in whatever form that may take, we find that healing happens wherever we go. Other people simply benefit from our presence. Our very existence is an act of healing. In this way we can have a much more powerful and often profound impact on the world around us than we would otherwise. To practice Reiki, we need to begin to respond to our own innate disposition to unfold towards wholeness.

In 2009 I went to a talk in Oxford, England, given by the Dalai Lama. I was fortunate enough to have a seat close to where His Holiness would enter the arena, so I had a very good view. For half an hour I sat there feeling very happy to be at such an event and excited for the opportunity to see and listen to one of the world's great spiritual teachers. Suddenly there was the sound of bells and chanting and monks started to file in followed by the Dalai Lama with more monks following on from behind. It was all very colorful and quite exotic. Then the Dalai Lama walked past where I was seated. As he did so great waves of peace seemed to ripple outwards from the center of his being. I felt a deep and profound sense of calm, connectivity, serenity and contentment simply by being in his presence. But what was going on? Why was I having what can only be described as a healing experience? My experience of being in his presence was not unusual of course, I'm sure that many people have experienced something similar, nor is it an experience that is confined to spiritual teachers in the Buddhist tradition. This type of experience happens on a regular basis with great teachers in all traditions the world over. Such teachers do not engage in their practice so that they might go around doing hands-on healing to one individual after another. The simple fact is that their very presence brings healing. Healing is a consequence of their being in the world. This is precisely what we should be aspiring to in our own daily practice. If you want to heal the world, work on yourself and the world will follow.

Of course, if you wish to focus your work with Reiki on using it as a hands-on therapy this is a perfectly fine thing to do and many people can benefit from your skills in this area. There is no "right way" with Reiki. Mikao Usui's system, however, (as opposed to the system that sprung from it, created by his student Chujiro Hayashi, which is what the world is largely practicing under Usui's name), is a powerful alchemical method for the transformation of the raw materials of the human condition into a more rarefied and pure state of being. To use it as such, whether we are focused on being a Reiki therapist or on our own journey of liberation, we cannot rely on just one aspect of the method (hands-on healing). This leaves us profoundly out of balance and really going nowhere very interesting very quickly (other than down the long dark tunnel of the ego). We need to engage with mindfulness meditation, too, and this should be a critical priority. Mindfulness is, as we have seen, the release-valve into awareness at the core of the Reiki experience. We need to endeavor to bring our mindfulness practice into every aspect of our daily lives not just into those moments where we consider ourselves to be engaged in spiritual practice, and we can support that process with hands-on healing. There is a powerful symbiotic relationship between the expansive awareness of reality that arises from mindfulness and the intense engagement with rarefied states of being that arises out of self-applications of spiritual energy. But just how do we bring all this spiritual practice into our everyday moment to moment existence? How do we break down those artificial barriers between what we consider to be "spiritual practice" and those times when we're immersed in what we believe to be our normal, everyday "non-spiritual" lives?

Firstly, we have those times when we are involved in what we could call our "formal" practice: when we sit on our cushion or mat or chair in a well composed meditation posture, which is our chance for some intensive practice. It's an opportunity to bring our focus and awareness fully to the task at hand and take our practice to a deeper level. But it's important to note as we engage in this practice what psychologist Christopher Germer pointed out in his book *The Mindful Path to Self-Compassion*: "The purpose of sitting... is to transform your daily life, not to get into altered states of consciousness[1]" and we really do need to keep this in mind. The practice of Reiki whether in its transference-of-energy aspect, or in its meditational aspect is not about gaining incredible psychic abilities to impress your friends. It's about improving the quality of your ordinary day to day existence as well as the lives of others. The most effective plan of action therefore is to have both a formal (sitting in meditation) and an informal (what we do in the rest of our lives off the cushion) practice. These two components or different approaches will support each other in a deep way. How we organize our practice is of course dependent on our own individual life circumstances, but certainly we should be aware of those times in our lives when we are in need and could benefit from the support that we can give to ourselves. If we are feeling discomfort or ill at ease in some way, we should take a moment out of our day to spend a few moments to at least bring some loving kindness to ourselves. What is wonderful about the practice of loving kindness in a Reiki context is that it can take the form of both a meditative activity and as a transmission of pure loving kindness energetically via the hands (or indeed, directly from the heart). So, we should be maximising our use of this ability as much as we can. We all need more love in our lives!

We should not be complacent, however, once we have committed to our practice and have started to reap some of the benefits. We are human beings and prone to falling back into time-worn habits and ways of being. Even if we gain spiritual insights and experience major openings in our awareness, at some point we will experience situations that once more trigger our emotions or bring our deep psychological issues to the surface. For most of us the reality is that our spiritual practices will only scratch the surface of our conditioned personality. The version of the "self" that we have formed and carry around with us stays largely undisturbed by our endeavors to unseat the ego and to realise full spiritual awakening. But this is okay. There are no rules that say we must achieve a state of perfection, enlightenment or permanently recline within the bliss of nirvana as quickly as possible so that we may say that we have succeeded in our spiritual practice. If we can be aware just for one moment, this is success enough. And then we work on the next moment, and then the next. The moments are endless, as can be our awareness of them. We just need to be willing to engage with the base practice of mindfulness meditation alongside the abundant flow of the subtle energy within and without us.

One way we can start to make inroads into impacting on our conditioned everyday relationship with life is by doing something called the Three Minute Breathing Space (3MBS).[2] The Three Minute Breathing Space is taking our practice of mindfulness out of our formal setting and applying it to our everyday moment to moment lives, especially those times when our automatic pilot might have taken over. There are basically three aspects to the practice of 3MBS, each lasting for approximately one minute:

Attending to what is happening right now. In this stage we simply note whatever arises and comes into our awareness in the present moment. It is a wide-open state that is free from decision-making or choices or any kind of judgment and we are not trying to change anything. We simply allow whatever arises to arise in our consciousness and we stay with it for about a minute. We are just watching each experience from one moment to the next.

Bringing awareness to the breath. We now bring our open awareness of our wider experiences down into a much narrower, single-pointed or concentrated focus on the breath. We find one place in the body where we can be aware of the experience of breathing, for instance, in the belly, or the chest or at the nose, or even in our back or the pelvic floor. Wherever we become conscious of the impact of the breath, we can keep our attention at that point in a narrow focus. Again, we stay here for one minute.

Bringing awareness to the whole body. In this final step we open out our awareness once more to include the whole body and the breath, noting any sensations that might be present. This last phase also takes about a minute.

The 3MBS is a way of taking a break from your daily routine, mindfully. The practice was developed by Zindel Segal, John Teasdale and Mark Williams for the MBCT (Mindfulness Based Cognitive Therapy) program and was described beautifully by way of an analogy in *The Mindful Way through Depression* co-authored with Jon Kabat-Zinn. Here is the difference between just taking a break and taking a breathing space:

> *Most of us have at some time been caught in a severe downpour and have had to run for shelter, perhaps in a shop doorway. Sometimes we are simply glad to be out of the rain. We stand for a while, hoping it will stop. We are dry at the moment, but as the rain continues, we know that sooner or later we are going to have to face it; the thing we tried to escape is still here. Finally, in one scenario, we go back out into the rain, grumbling, even cursing our luck as the rain drenches us.*
>
> *At other times, another scenario might unfold for us. We may take shelter in a very different way. We stand in a doorway for a while, aware of the prospect of getting soaked and not liking it much. We notice that we are hoping that it will stop but, seeing that it shows no sign of stopping realise that being upset about it and worrying about how soaked we are going to get is only adding to our discomfort. So, we stop clinging to the hope that it will stop raining and enter the downpour, letting ourselves be drenched and accepting that this is what is happening at the moment. Approaching the situation in this way may allow us to experience the rain itself. We may notice that there is something rather compelling about the way it is splashing off everything it hits. The rain has not stopped. We may be getting wetter and wetter.*

But our relationship to what is happening has changed the whole experience. (Williams et al., 2009)[3]

The 3MBS helps to provide a structure for reclaiming our sense of ease and centeredness at those times when situations in life might be quite challenging or when we have reverted to our automatic pilot and are just missing everything! The 3MBS allows us to approach reality from both a wide and a narrow perspective in a very short timeframe, the effect of which starts to seep more and more into all of our everyday activities.

Here is a Three Minute Breathing Space meditation for you to practice which you should attempt to do several times a day and especially at those times when life seems to be spiralling out of control. The practice given here is set up as a formal meditation practice, but at those times when you don't have your meditation cushion with you, you can do this practice standing or walking anywhere that you happen to be. Set a timer on your phone and just stop right where you are and do the practice once an hour or every couple of hours. Even a couple of times a day is beneficial. The idea is to integrate mindfulness more and more into our lives.

Three Minute Breathing Space

First of all, assume your meditation posture and get comfortable, making sure that your hands are resting comfortably in your lap. You may close your eyes or if you wish you can focus on a spot on the wall or the floor in front of you. Cultivate a sense of openness and expansiveness in the chest area, and if necessary, place your hands on a cushion to facilitate this. Now settle into your posture, allowing your shoulders to release all tension on each out breath. Check that your spine is straight, resting into its natural curve. Sitting forward of the back of the chair if you are using a chair for this meditation but supporting your back with a cushion if necessary. Check that your head is nicely balanced, the crown supporting the sky. Feel a sense of quiet dignity about yourself, how you are sat, and your state of mind.

Now take a couple of slightly deeper breaths than normal and bring yourself fully into the present moment. Notice whatever it is that you are experiencing right now. Be aware of any sensations that you might be experiencing. Be aware of your feet on the ground, your connection to the chair or cushion or the floor. Notice the sensation of your clothes against your body and the air against your skin. Now notice any thoughts that are passing through your mind. Whatever thoughts come up, just observe them with clarity and without letting them drag you into their story, remind yourself that thoughts are not facts. Thoughts are simply mental events playing out across the endless expanse of your mind. Be aware of whatever you are feeling emotionally and notice where those emotions might be impacting on your body, in particular any unpleasant or uncomfortable feelings and allow yourself to turn towards them, acknowledging their presence. Don't try to change your emotions, just allow them to be, and rest in awareness of them. If there are any physical sensations of discomfort or tension just allow yourself to become aware of them, noting whatever is in this moment.

Bring your attention to your breath. Be aware of the movement of the abdomen, the rise and fall of your belly as you breathe in and out. Every time your mind wanders, just note it and gently bring it back to rest on the breath. Feel the coolness of each in breath and the warmth of each out breath. Notice the passing of each breath as it gives way to the rising of the next breath. Each breath is like a wave on an ocean, rising and falling and then another wave, another breath, rising and falling. Bind your awareness to the rise and fall of each breath.

Now expand your awareness to feel the breath moving throughout your body, allowing for a more spacious awareness of your experience. Feel where the body is responding to the breath, allowing your experience of the breath to just rest in the background of your awareness. Do you notice the breath in your back, in your belly, your chest, maybe you can sense it as an echo down in the pelvic floor?

Notice your whole body, from head to toe. Bring your awareness to your thinking process and whatever emotions are present for you right now. Allow your awareness to expand outwards, to broaden, noticing all aspects of your experience, holding everything in your awareness.

Now slowly bring your attention back to the room that you are in. Feel your connection to the earth through your feet and gently and in your own time, open your eyes. Just take a moment to let your surroundings sink in; what you can see, what you can hear. Allow yourself to stretch before resuming your daily activities.

Working regularly with the 3MBS will certainly help to integrate mindfulness into your daily life and help to embed it into any energy healing work that you might engage in. There are other ways that you can also begin to integrate mindfulness into your daily life, however. One such approach is something called the Habit Releaser.

Habit Releasers

Habit Releasers can help to break down and release us from the automatic pilot that has taken over the navigation of so much of our lives. Whether it's brushing our teeth, shaving, brushing our hair or even driving the car, so much of life is done in automaton mode. We are not present. Deliberately intervening in our habitual responses to life can reignite our passion and curiosity and bring us home to the moment. A Habit Releaser can be something very simple. For instance, noticing which chair you sit in at meetings at work or to watch TV in the evening and deliberately choosing to sit in a different chair (be careful not to upset someone else by sitting in their chair!). Maybe you could drive a different route to work for a change or go to the park and walk barefoot on the grass, even if it's raining! It would be worthwhile practicing each Habit Releaser for a few days before changing it. Try not to stick with it for so long that it simply becomes a new habit, however.

Here are some other Habit Releasers you might try:

Brush your teeth with the opposite hand. If we use a different hand to brush our teeth, we suddenly find that we need to be a lot more present with the activity. Notice the texture and movement of the brush, the sensation on the teeth and gums, how the brush feels in the hand, the movement of the arm all the way up to the shoulder.

Watch a kettle boil. When I was doing my mindfulness meditation training with Breathworks,[4] I really got into this Habit Releaser and it's still one of my favorites. My personal mentor during my training didn't like this one at all! You can make up your own mind. Pick up the kettle, noting its weight and how it feels in the hand and fill it, mindfully. Place it down and flick the switch. Close your eyes and just be present with the sound of the kettle as it boils. One time I did this practice I was leaning with both hands on the work surface that the kettle sat on. As it boiled, I could feel the subtle vibrations that were set up by the boiling kettle rippling through the work surface under my hands. There is a lot to focus on in this Habit Releaser.

Try a different brand of chocolate. If you are going to buy chocolate or any other type of confectionary, why not try something you have never tried before, or one that you haven't eaten recently? It could be an expensive and sophisticated brand, or it might be something cheap and trashy. Open it up and first of all inhale the aroma. Really notice how the smell impacts deep inside. Where is it reaching? Break off a piece and feel its texture. When you place it in your mouth, can you hold it there for a few moments and really notice what it feels like? Can you pick out any of the distinct flavors?

Standing in a line. If you find yourself having to queue somewhere, this is a perfect opportunity to practice mindfulness. Life doesn't get any better than this in terms of mindfulness opportunities! Feel the contact with the floor through your feet. Notice how your body feels, be aware of any sensations that might be present. Notice how your center of gravity shifts, feeling the weight of your body. Are there any sensations or feelings of stress or impatience anywhere in the body? Notice these also.

Listening. Can you listen to someone without falling into agreeing or disagreeing with them? Can you be attentive in the moment without planning what you are going to say in response? Can you be with their words fully without creating your own mental commentary about what they are saying?

Random acts of kindness. We all appreciate it when someone is kind to us. This is an opportunity for you to do some small act that could improve or benefit another person's life in some way. If you are feeling especially bold and you want to develop your *metta* practice in some practical way, you could perhaps try to do something for someone that you find a little difficult or even dislike. Try to do this with no expectation of return, however. The benefit is in the giving, not in what you might receive back. You could even do this random act anonymously. Perhaps you could buy a friend their coffee or pay the bill for someone else in a coffee shop or restaurant. There are many ways in which we can be more kind to each other.

Go for a walk. What time is your favorite soap on TV? Why not go for a walk at that time instead and try to put out of your mind what you might (but actually won't) be missing with your characters in the TV show? Be present with where you are, the touch of the air on your skin, the feel or sound of your footsteps. Notice the sounds all around you. Is it raining or sunny? Windy? Snowing? Be with whatever experience life is presenting to you right in this moment. If you regularly go for a walk anyway, why not walk somewhere different?

There are dozens of ways we can take the normal activities of everyday life and tweak them so that we can seize them from the clutches of the automatic pilot and more easily bring mindfulness into our lives. The whole point of these activities is to slowly make more and more of our lives mindful. A mindful life is infinitely more valuable and joyful than a mindless one. Developing mindfulness of daily life is also absolutely central to developing your practice of Reiki as a personal spiritual development system and also as an energy-based therapy.

When you are working in a hands-on capacity with another human being, you owe it to your client to be utterly present in the moment for them. Whether working with a pre-defined set of hand positions or working intuitively with a sophisticated understanding of the nature of the movement of energy (*Byosen*), it is important to be aware and utterly detached in your practice. When you are giving a treatment, you are in the act of sensing the energy directly with your hands (and possibly with your eyes or inner vision), both within the body of the client and in your own hands. The depth of penetration of the energy into the body of the client is predicated on your ability to focus and flow with your experience of the moment. You may feel warmth, tingling, vibration or some indefinable sensation, all of which can arise and surge and change their nature and then recede within the frame of your awareness. The observer changes that which is observed, so it's important to be still, empty, void-like. When you stand to treat, do Standing Meditation, when you sit, do Sitting Meditation. Keep bringing your mind back to stillness. Keep your mind off the idea of transmitting energy. The energy doesn't need you. Just stand or sit with your client and practice Reiki. This is Qigong: two *Qi* fields interacting with one another and tending towards oneness. The depth and quality of the healing experience is related to the depth of awareness and stillness of the practitioner.

Practicing mindfulness meditation is a liberating experience. Practicing Reiki is a liberating experience, but whereas mindfulness exists as a discrete discipline, there is no Reiki without mindfulness. Without mindfulness what is left of Reiki is a pale shadow of what it might have been.

You don't need to want to achieve enlightenment in your spiritual practice, whatever that practice may be. You just need to want to be a better human being and if you can achieve that, you have achieved a lot. In the end, all you need to do is flow. Form is emptiness, emptiness is form, and Reiki is the subtle energy-wind that weaves through them and binds them together.

Afterword

Some time ago as a very ordinary morning meditation came to an end, the words of Shunryū Suzuki suddenly came to mind; when we sit to meditate with the intention of doing something special, we are doing nothing at all. They morphed out of abstraction into a vibrantly alive conscious experience that completely stunned me. Two bells on my phone had just bonged to mark the end of the meditation and I sat for a moment readying myself for the start of the day. The morning's meditation had been characterised by the usual scuttling of random thoughts, interspersed with fleeting moments of awareness and focus. There were also, from what I recall, occasional digressions into blissful stillness which are always amazing when they happen, but they are moments that generally tend to evaporate as soon as you look at them, giving way to another train of thoughts of largely no consequence.

On this day, just as I gave up the meditation, I felt a very subtle shift in my awareness. It was like when you walk in the door with two heavy shopping bags and can finally put them down: a moment of relief as you feel the tension go out of you. You relax a little, perhaps sigh and maybe think about making a cup of tea. The effort of carrying the bags… of the meditation now all finished. At that moment, as I gave up on meditating, I felt a deep stillness, almost a sense of merging with my breath which, curiously, a few moments before I had been struggling to stay focused on. This reaction is actually very common amongst Western meditators who tend to strive in their meditation in an effort to achieve something – let's say, reducing stress – thus unwittingly blocking the spaciousness and stillness that was always there, just behind all that striving. When we can simply sit in a state of open awareness, insight can spontaneously arise which then has the knock-on-effect of reducing such things as stress in any case. This tends to happen as we become more familiar with the workings of the mind and its reactions to the various senses and the world around us.

Suzuki's words had had a profound impact on me long ago when I'd first read *Zen Mind, Beginners Mind*. I was familiar with the idea of just being natural on the cushion; not doing anything special and just sitting to sit. When a frog is a frog, Zen is Zen, as the saying goes. But here I was, emerging from a meditation, like so many meditations before it, where, unbeknownst to me, I had fallen hook, line and sinker for the trap laid by my ego. I was being special. I was being a Meditator, and I hadn't even noticed it. This is like the frog trying its best to be a frog. All it had to do was to stop trying to be a frog and just be a frog!

We need to realise that the ego is just as smart as we are. There is no getting away from this. It can hijack our spiritual practice, our Reiki practice, just as surely as night follows day and you won't even notice it. So, how can we put the methods described in this book to use in a meaningful way without them getting subverted by the machinations of the ego? One solution to this is to look at a practice called "On Duty, Off Duty." It's a practice that was taught by Khenpo Lhabu at Samye Ling monastery in Scotland.[1]

On Duty, Off Duty is a practice that is designed to enable a practitioner to more easily find the right balance between focused and open awareness, but I think it also has a great deal to offer in enabling us to cut down our predisposition towards "trying to meditate" which is the bane of so many of us in the West. It's a practice that works by alternating through three-minute periods of meditation and then rest from meditation. The On Duty part is when you are meditating. Here we can follow the breath (such as in the Breathing Anchor meditation) or meditate on the symbols and explore the methods and develop the skills that sensitise us in our practice. The Off Duty part is when we have stopped meditating and are sat at rest, doing nothing.

This is how it works, and you can apply it to every one of the meditations in this book:

On Duty, Off Duty

Set a timer on your mobile phone to go off every three minutes. Sit and do your meditation: focusing on your breath or visualising the Reiki symbols in your inner vision or sending out metta to all beings everywhere. Whatever meditation you wish to work with is fine.

When the timer goes off, stop your meditation. You are now Off Duty. If your eyes were closed, open them. You can look around if you wish but try not to have a sense of wanting to do something or engage with anything. If any thoughts arise, this is perfectly fine. See if you can rest into a sense of spaciousness.

When the timer goes off, go back On Duty. When you are On Duty acknowledge whatever happens with your mind and say "yes" to whatever arises. Whatever it is, it's okay. Allow and accept whatever the mind does. This will help encourage the quality of spaciousness more, allowing it to manifest within the On Duty periods.

If thoughts do arise, you can if you wish, try to backtrack to the previous thought and the one before that, and identify the original thought that started the train in motion. Perhaps see if you can sit with that original thought and observe it. What does it feel like? Where does it rest in the body?

Keep repeating the On Duty, Off Duty process for as long as you wish. Remember that, at least for Western meditators, the one thing that seems to block meditation the most is the act of trying to meditate.

The main thing is to enjoy your practice. There is nothing to achieve, nowhere to go. Reiki and meditation are not enlightenment projects.

May all beings be happy.

Some further thoughts

In writing this book I have attempted to stay as close to the known historical information regarding the development, philosophy and methodology of the system of Reiki as I can. After a period of time in the early days of Reiki's expansion in the West during the 1990s and early part of the new millennium, the system was being profoundly corrupted by all manner of ad hoc New Age additions. Extra symbols, the inclusion of such things as "Reiki Guides" (spirit guides), understandings and practices imported from various energy healing disciplines and other therapies and highly dubious "channeled" material of various kinds were being thrown into the Reiki melting pot, diluting it and turning it into a system that was and still is widely ridiculed. In reaction to that there has been, quite understandably, a growing "purist" approach to the system, whereby pretty much everything that doesn't have its origins in Japan and Japanese spirituality is being jettisoned.

I believe that there needs to be some balance brought to this. It is known that the founder of Reiki, Mikao Usui, traveled widely prior to his development of the system. It is also known that we don't know everything about what exactly he learnt on those travels or what teachings and practices he drew on in the formulation of his system. What we do know is that he seems to have drawn heavily on esoteric Buddhist practices, most likely those that inform a Japanese understanding of Buddhist practice. However, esoteric Buddhism in Japan has an equivalence in Tibetan esoteric Buddhism: many practices, if not identical, differ only in as much as they have a slightly different cultural context and flavor. Whilst at the present time, no evidence has emerged for the precise teachings within Japanese esoteric Buddhism that Usui might have drawn on, there are teachings held within the lineage of Reiki Jin Kei Do, with a distinctly Tibetan origin, that suggest very clearly and very heavily that Usui almost certainly accessed those teachings, if not in their

Tibetan form, then most likely in their Japanese equivalent. What is very clear is that as time has gone on, new research and new understandings of Reiki's origins have inexorably been moving very powerfully in the direction of the teachings that have been held within Reiki Jin Kei Do all along. The linkages between those teachings and modern secular Reiki are so profoundly obvious and so deeply intertwined with every aspect of the known Reiki system that it is inconceivable that there is not some direct relationship between the two.

If the system of Reiki is to be given the recognition that it deserves as a meaningful and incredibly rich spiritual development practice, surely it must distance itself not only from the many New Age aberrations but also avoid disappearing down the purist rabbit hole. A more expansive and open engagement with Reiki's possibilities, as well as its possible historical antecedents is necessary, it seems to me.

When you step into the zone of love, language as we know it becomes obsolete. That which cannot be put into words can only be grasped through silence.

Elif Shafak – *The Forty Rules of Love*

About the Author

Steve has been a regular freelance writer on the subjects of Reiki and mindfulness meditation for the past 30 years, contributing to journals and magazines in the UK and the Middle East. He has been teaching Reiki and meditation in the UK, Egypt, Sudan, Lithuania, Cyprus and Jordan since 1997 and regularly receives invitations to teach in other parts of the world. Since 2014, he has been teaching *Buddho*: the ancient Buddhist practice from which modern secular Reiki was derived. As a certified Breathworks teacher of mindfulness meditation, Steve delivers training to individuals and corporates across the UK. Breathworks is one of the world's lead bodies in the research and application of mindfulness meditation for health.

Steve is also a noted artist with work in collections around the world and loves spending time in art galleries and museums whenever the opportunity arises.

He has a passion for good literature, especially Arabic and American with occasional forays into Japanese and English literature. He also devours books on esoteric Buddhism along with classic French, English and American movies from the Golden Age of cinema.

Unusually for a teacher of Reiki, he has no real desire to travel to Japan on the well-worn Reiki pilgrimage route. But who knows what the future may bring?

Previous Titles

Reiki Jin Kei Do: The Way of Compassion & Wisdom

Set to fundamentally reshape the way that we think about Reiki as a healing method, this book is a must read for anyone seriously interested in this unique path to self-perfection and liberation. In the tradition of Reiki Jin Kei Do the emphasis of practice is on leading the student to a realization of their oneness and ultimate reunification with all-that-is. For the first time, all of the extant knowledge on the history of Reiki is in key figures pulled together. From Mikao Usui's enlightenment experience whilst practicing the Buddho meditation on Mt Kurama to the journey of the enigmatic Zen monk Seiji Takamori, high into the Himalayas of Nepal in search of Reiki's origins. Reiki Jin Kei Do (the way of compassion and wisdom through Reiki) contains the secret Indian/Tibetan teachings that Takamori received from the recluse monks with whom he studied. These teachings were passed on as the system now known as Buddho-EnerSense.

Steve Gooch offers a clear and concise understanding of the practice of Reiki, whilst illustrating the essential teachings of Reiki Jin Kei Do. This book is not only an engaging read, it also explains the Reiki symbols, Jin Kei Do meditations and methods for treating oneself and others. Whether you are new to Reiki or a seasoned practitioner, Reiki Jin Kei Do will be of tremendous benefit to anyone interested in this unique and wholesome style of Reiki.
Lawrence Ellyard, author of *Reiki Meditations* and *Reiki Healer*

A detailed, clear and fascinating insight into the world of Reiki. Excellent for beginners and particularly relevant to experienced

practitioners looking to expand their understanding and experience of Reiki.
David Vennells, author of *Reiki Mastery* and *Reiki for Beginners*

Revealing the Vajrayana and Tantric Buddhist origins of Reiki for the first time, this book will broaden the way you view Reiki, explaining it not simply as a healing system, but as a way of self-perfection and liberation which did not suddenly appear in the nineteenth century, but has a far older lineage.
Cygnus Books

A Message from the Author

I hope that you have enjoyed reading my book on mindfulness meditation and Reiki and perhaps found it to be of some benefit in how you engage with your own practice, whether that be in Reiki and/or mindfulness meditation.

If you have a few moments, please feel free to add a review of the book to your favorite online site.

If you feel motivated to explore mindfulness meditation further or to deepen your connection to the origins of Reiki and want to really explore "how," "what," and "why" this system has the relatively unexplored potential that it has, then feel free to check out my website at: www.omahhum.co where, when time allows, I post blogs, videos and other material related to the practice. You will also find a growing range of online and in person courses for you to attend to deepen your practice (mainly in the field of mindfulness meditation, which is my primary focus), and if you're a center anywhere in the world and want me to come and teach, for sure, please message me. You can contact me directly via the website.

With best wishes and much metta,

Steve Gooch, Cairo, Egypt, January 2021

Endnotes

Introduction

1 Quoted in Dyer, W. (2005). *You'll See It When You Believe It*, London, Arrow Books, page 64.

Chapter 1

1 Frank Arjava Petter's *Reiki Fire* (Twin Lakes, Lotus Light Publications) sent a shock wave through the world of Western Reiki when it was first published in 1997. It revealed for the first time aspects of the system, its philosophy and practice that had until then remained exclusively in Japan. Many of the basic understandings that the worldwide Reiki community had about the system turned out not to be so, or at best had been misunderstood or misinterpreted.

2 Quote from Taggart King's 2001 *Japanese Reiki Techniques* manual for students.

3 Following the publication of Frank Petter's ground-breaking books, Hiroshi Doi, a Japanese Reiki Master published a book in English called *Iyashi Gendai Reiki-ho: Modern Reiki Method of Healing* (Coquitlam, Fraser Journal Pub) in 2000, which again profoundly changed the world's understanding of the system of Reiki. Following this in 2005, *The Art of Japanese Reiki* (Ropley, O Books) by Bronwen and Frans Stiene sent yet another seismic shock wave through the world of Reiki.

4 See Frans Stiene's work in *The Inner Heart of Reiki: Rediscovering Your True Self* (Winchester, Ayni Books) to get a feel for the direction that current research into the system is going.

5 Taggart King, *Mindfulness and Compassion in Reiki Healing*: *https://www.reiki-evolution.co.uk/mindfulness-and-compassion/*

6 Quote from: *https://www.mindful.org/what-is-mindfulness/*

This is a good resource for information on mindfulness and with practices you can do at home.

7 If you wish to explore the use of mindfulness in healthcare settings, you can check out the Breathworks website. Breathworks are one of the world's lead bodies in the research and development of the use of mindfulness in healthcare settings, and are working with the UK's National Health Service: *https://www.breathworks-mindfulness.org.uk/*

8 Dr Danny Penman, *Mindfulness for Creativity,* London, Piatkus, pages 3 and 12–15.

9 Dr Mark Williams quoted on the NHS website at: *https://www.nhs.uk/conditions/stress-anxiety-depression/mindfulness/#*

10 Ed Halliwell, *Mindfulness: How to Live Well by Paying Attention,* London, Hay House, page 99.

11 Vessantara, *The Art of Meditation: The Breath,* Cambridge, Windhorse Publications, page 38.

12 Shunryū Suzuki, *Zen Mind, Beginners Mind,* Boulder, Shambhala Publications, Inc., page 11.

13 Karlfried Graf Durckheim, *Hara: The Vital Center of Man,* Rochester, Inner Traditions, page 166.

14 Shunryū Suzuki, *Zen Mind, Beginners Mind,* Boulder, Shambhala Publications, Inc., page 32.

Chapter 2

1 For a good retelling of the history of Reiki and Dr Usui's life, refer to Frank Petter's *This Is Reiki* (Twin Lakes, Lotus Press) or Penelope Quest's *Reiki for Life* (London, Piatkus), (Quest's book includes an early and erroneous Christianised telling of the history of Reiki, which is amended by the author through a note to the text in later editions).

2 See Nicholas Pearson, *Foundations of Reiki Ryoho: A Manual of Shoden and Okuden,* Rochester, Healing Arts Press, pages 84–85 for further information.

3 There is a lot of disagreement over the accuracy of the

various translations of the Reiki Precepts that are available in various books and across the internet. It is my belief that it is most important to get to the true essence of a text rather than to simply give a *verbatim* transcription of the original. Skilled literary translators are highly prized in their field for their ability to strike the right balance between staying as true to the original text as possible and at the same time being able to apply artistic licence judiciously when it is necessary to change the precise word form of the original in order to convey its true essence. This is why I have chosen to discuss Frans Stiene's version in Chapter 2. Here is a more accurate translation of the Precepts by Dr Mark Hosak if you wish to compare it with Stiene's:

Secret method to invite happiness
Spiritual cure of countless diseases
Especially on this day – being angry – let go
Worries – let go
Be thankful
Take care of your karma
Be kind to all living creatures
In the morning and evening – put your hands together in front of your heart
Place your attention into your spiritual heart
Recite them with the mouth
Continuous improvement process for the body, mind and spiritual heart
Method of natural healing with spiritual life energy by Usui
Usui Mikao

4 Frans Stiene, *The Inner Heart of Reiki: Rediscovering Your True Self*, Winchester, Ayni Books, page 59.

5 Penelope Quest, *Reiki for Life: The Complete Guide to Reiki Practice for Levels 1, 2 and 3*, London, Piatkus, page 13.

6 The Pali language is the language of the early Therevadan Buddhist texts and believed to be the language that the

Buddha himself spoke. It died out in India as a literary language in the fourteenth century.

7 Frans Stiene, *The Inner Heart of Reiki: Rediscovering Your True Self,* Winchester, Ayni Books, page 45–46.

8 Quoted in Vidyamala Burch and Danny Penman, *Mindfulness for Health,* London, Piatkus, page 204.

9 Frank Petter was the first Western Reiki Master to bring some of the true historical information and original methods of Reiki to a Western audience. *The Three Pillars of Reiki* were introduced to the West as a concept by Petter in his book: *The Original Reiki Handbook of Dr. Mikao Usui,* (Twin Lakes, Lotus Press).

10 "Gassho literally means 'two hands coming together'" (Petter, 1999, page 15), but if we look a little deeper, as Frans Stiene has noted, *Gassho* is symbolic of non-duality. It is the coming together of two opposites; two things become one. "[M]orning and evening, one should perform Gassho, to remember one's non-dualistic nature" (Stiene, 2015, page 55). According to esoteric Buddhism, the left hand represents the moon, and the right hand represents the sun (Petter, 2001, page 148).

11 According to Wikipedia a *mudra* is "a spiritual gesture and an energetic seal of authenticity employed in the iconography and spiritual practice of Indian religions," such as in Hinduism, Buddhism and Jainism. *https://en.wikipedia.org/wiki/Mudra*

12 Karen Frazer wrote an excellent article on The Three Pillars of Reiki at *https://www.authorkarenfrazier.com/blog/engaging-in-the-flow-of-reiki-through-its-three-pillars* emphasising the need for a focused and mindful engagement with the practice, rather than a fairly short perfunctory practice of a moment or so.

13 If you are going to recite the Precepts or *Gokai* each day, then you should try reciting them in Japanese and also in

translation into your native language. Decide for yourself in which language you are most comfortable reciting them. When Muslims recite the Quran, they do so in classical Arabic, the Catholic Tridentine Mass is in Latin and Nichiren Buddhists chant the Daimoku in Japanese. Whether the secular Reiki Precepts contain *kotodama* (spiritual power) in the same way that these religious practices do, is a point that is open to debate. Reiki Master Tado Yamaguchi in his excellent book, *Light on the Origins of Reiki,* (Twin Lakes, Lotus Press – Shangri-La), page 93, commented on this and has made the claim that the Precepts do contain *kotodama*.

14 Frank Arvaja Petter, *This Is Reiki,* Twin Lakes, Lotus Press, pages 24–25.

15 Andrew Miller, *Japan's Modern Myth: The Language and Beyond,* New York & Tokyo, John Weatherhill, pages xii and 298.

Chapter 3

1 See Rick Rivard's comments on *The Reiki Threshold* at *http://www.threshold.ca/reiki/sample/index.html*

2 This idea of Reiki having different qualities or frequencies or vibrations that you could access through the various symbols, is a Western New Age addition to the system and one that is at odds with the way the symbols actually work. To quote James Deacon from his *Reiki Pages*: "as various forms of western Reiki were imported into Japan, this thoroughly modern, western 'New Age' perception of the symbols also found its way into the newly-evolving Japanese Reiki, and it was not long before we were being asked to believe that not only was this in fact an original Japanese perception, but that this was the primary reason why Usui-sensei had introduced the symbols into Reiki in the first place: to assist certain students in differentiating between the various different aspects or qualities – the

various 'energies within Reiki'...!!" *(https://www.aetw.org/reiki_symbols_more.htm#symb)*. What the symbols do is to connect the practitioner to different qualities or aspects of themselves.

3 Frans Stiene, *Reiki Insights,* Winchester, Ayni Books, pages 112 to 113.

4 There is a lot of controversy over the inclusion or even the slightest mention of the *chakras* in relation to Reiki. It's important to note that there is no reference to the *chakra* system at all in Japanese esoteric Buddhism (the principal origin of much of the Reiki system). This form of Buddhism arrived in Japan with the teacher Kukai. Kukai had studied in China and taken what he had learnt back to Japan where it evolved into a distinctly Japanese version of esoteric Buddhism. However, the main esoteric text in which the *chakras* are mentioned and utilised (Anuttarayoga Tantra) was not translated into Chinese until after Kukai's time. However, to assume that Symbol 1 has no relationship to the *chakra* system is to assume that it is solely derived from Japanese esoteric systems and cannot be found and is not utilised in any other cultural, religious or spiritual context. Esoteric symbols are not culturally specific and not "invented" within a culture. They are direct emanations of the culture-free universal energy field. It is also worth noting that it is known that Usui traveled to and studied in China. Can we speculate that it's possible he studied the Anuttarayoga Tantra whilst there?

5 Even as late as 2018, new Reiki books are appearing that use the *mantra* as the name of the symbol (Nicholas Pearson's *Foundations of Reiki Ryoho* [Rochester, Healing Arts Press] for instance). Somewhat confusingly, Tadao Yamaguchi in his *Light on the Origins of Reiki* (Twin Lakes, Lotus Press – Shangri-La) seems to imply that the *mantras* are also names and that *mantras* are repeated out loud, but names

are not (pages 140–141). For a better understanding of the relationship between the mantric and symbolic devices, check out Torsten Lange's *Reiki: Heal Your Body and Your Life with the Power of Universal Energy,* (London: Hay House), or the latter work of Frans Stiene *(Reiki Insights* and *The Inner Heart of Reiki* [Winchester, Ayni Books]).

6 Frank Arjava Petter, *Reiki Fire,* Twin Lakes, Lotus Light Publications, page 110.

7 Bronwen and Frans Stiene, *The Japanese Art of Reiki,* Ropley, O Books, page 123 and associated note on page 187.

8 James Deacon, *James Deacon's Reiki Pages*: *http://www.aetw.org/reiki_symbols2.html*

9 Hiroshi Doi, *Iyashi Gendai Reiki-ho: Modern Reiki Method for Healing,* Coquitlam, Fraser Journal Publishing, page 146.

10 A *Bodhisattva* is "a person who has achieved great moral and spiritual wisdom and is a potential Buddha, esp. such a person who rejects nirvana in order to assist suffering mankind." See: *https://www.yourdictionary.com/Bodhisattva*

11 Don Beckett, *Reiki, the True Story,* Berkeley, Frog Books, page 119.

12 Nicholas Pearson, *Foundations of Reiki Ryoho,* Rochester, Healing Arts Press, pages 239–242.

13 Nicholas Pearson, *Foundations of Reiki Ryoho,* Rochester, Healing Arts Press, page 241.

14 From a personal communication with Mark Hosak.

15 You can find *A Practice of Transference Involving Amitbha* here: *https://static.squarespace.com/static/50be4fefe4b0c82b6072c4ed/t/53691321e4b0b561109cff5a/1399395105551/amitabha.pdf* and *"The Practice Called Opening the Eye"* here: *https://shop.fpmt.org/Prayer-to-Chenrezig-Compassionate-Eye-Looking-One-PDF_p_3137.html*

16 An excellent book on the tantric practices of using *mantra* and *yantra* is *Tools for Tantra* (Vermont, Destiny Books), by Harish Johari.

17 Quote from Madhu Khanna, *Yantra: The Tantric Symbol of Cosmic Unity*, (London, Thames & Hudson), page 34.

18 It has been claimed that Symbol 1 can be found in Tendai cosmology and is connected to an old Japanese text called Hotsuma Tsutae: an elaborate epic poem of Japanese legendary history and apparently used by Tendai Priests (see *The Japanese Art of Reiki* [Ropley, O Books], page 124 and *The Reiki Sourcebook* [Winchester, O Books], pages 90–92, both books by Bronwen and Frans Stiene). The document is controversial and many leading academics in Japan consider it to be a fake (For an analysis of the Hotsuma Tutsae, see *What's Hotsuma Tutsae?* here: *https://japanophilia.xyz/2018/06/06/hotsuma-tsutae/*). From this text was developed the Hotsumani Futomani Divination Chart (you can find a copy of the chart here: *http://hotsuma.gr.jp/futomani-e.html*), which contains two spirals representing "heaven" and "earth" (*a* and *wa*); which are the supposed origin of Symbol 1. However, they are just spirals and no more visually close to Symbol 1 than any other spiral. It has also been claimed that Symbol 1 has an origin in Taoism, but this has not been verified (see *The Reiki Sourcebook* by Bronwen and Frans Stiene, page 91 and another claim made by Reiki Master Dave King in relation to a set of notes given to him by one of Chujiro Hayashi's students; Tatsumi, which makes the claim for all of the symbols appearing in the *Daozang* [a collection of texts on Taoism, including all the commentaries and expositions of various masters in an attempt to pull together all the extant material on Taoist teachings]. See *Reiki, the True Story* [Berkeley, Frog Books] by Don Beckett, page 119). If the symbol does appear within Taoism, as some have suggested, it is most likely due to it being absorbed into the Taoist canon after the arrival of Buddhism in China and given Usui's involvement at a very deep level with the practice of *Qigong*, perhaps this is

where he first encountered it. According to author Nicholas Pearson in *Foundations of Reiki Ryoho*, (Rochester, Healing Arts Press), Symbol 1 has its roots in Shintoism (pages 228–229). Again, there is no evidence for this, but as esoteric Buddhism mixed with Shinto practices on its arrival and subsequent development in Japan, it is possible that the symbol, originally Buddhist, ended up being absorbed into Shinto.

19 Bronwen and Frans Stiene, *The Reiki Sourcebook*, Winchester, O Books, page 92; James Deacon, *James Deacon's Reiki Pages*: *http://www.aetw.org/reiki_symbolsP.html*

20 Bronwen and Frans Stiene, *The Reiki Sourcebook,* Winchester, O Books, page 92. Another name for Seishi is Vajrapani. The *vajra* that Seishi/Vajrapani wields has great significance to the development of the Reiki system.

21 James Deacon, *The Reiki Symbols – Ongoing Research* which can be downloaded here: *http://www.aetw.org/reiki_pdf.htm*

22 James Deacon, *The Reiki Symbols – Ongoing Research* which can be downloaded here: *http://www.aetw.org/reiki_pdf.htm*

23 Quote in Jojan Jonker, *Reiki: The Transmigration of a Japanese Spiritual Healing Practice,* Zurich, Lit Verlag, page 408 from an interview by Stein and Hirano with Yoshie Kimura; one of the students on Mrs Takata's very first Reiki class in Hilo, Hawaii.

24 Quoted from *Zen Mind, Beginners Mind,* Boulder, Shambhala Publications, Inc, by Shunryū Suzuki, page 34.

25 Frank Petter, *This Is Reiki,* Twin Lakes, Lotus Press, page 153.

26 There are five Buddha families: the Buddha family, the Vajra Family, the Ratna Family, the Lotus Family and the Karma Family.

27 *Om Ah Hum* is also the *mantra* of the Buddhas of the Three Times: the Buddha of the past: Dipamkara, the Buddha of the future: Maitreya and the Buddha of the present: Shakyamuni.

28 Sogyal Rinpoche, *The Tibetan Book of Living and Dying*, London, Rider, pages 386–387. *Dharmakaya, Sambhogakaya* and *Nirmanakaya* are The Three *Kayas (Trikaya)* that exist in Mahayana and Vajrayana Buddhism.

29 A good basic guide to Dainichi Buddha can be found in *Shingon Esoteric Buddhism: A Handbook for Followers*, Fresno, Shingon Buddhist International Institute, page 66 or for a more thorough understanding, check out Vessantara's *Meeting the Buddhas: A Guide to Buddhas, Bodhisattvas, and Tantric Deities,* Birmingham, Windhorse Publications, Chapter 10.

30 *http://soundofom.com/om/*

31 A good basic outline of what *kanji* are all about and how they developed, can be found here: *https://www.nihongomaster.com/blog/what-is-kanji/*

32 Nicholas Pearson, *Foundations of Reiki Ryoho,* Rochester, Healing Arts Press, page 251.

33 Nicholas Pearson, *Foundations of Reiki Ryoho,* Rochester, Healing Arts Press, page 252.

34 Mark Hosak's, Walter Lubeck, *The Big Book of Reiki Symbols,* Twin Lakes, Lotus Press, page 344.

35 See Encyclopaedia Britannica: *https://www.britannica.com/topic/stupa*

36 James Deacon, *James Deacon's Reiki Pages*: *http://www.aetw.org/reiki_symbolsD.html*

37 Frans Stiene, *The Inner Heart of Reiki,* Winchester, Ayni Books, page 77.

38 Steve Gooch, *Reiki Jin Kei Do Level 2 manual*, 1997.

39 James Deacon, *James Deacon's Reiki Pages*: *http://www.aetw.org/reiki_symbolsD.html*. This is a really interesting point and I often point out to my students that the system of Reiki is essentially all self-treatment. When we talk about treating another person, it is just another aspect or way of looking at self-treatment, as there is no "other" to give a treatment to.

40 Frans Stiene, *The Inner Heart of Reiki,* Winchester, Ayni Books, page 78.

41 Bronwen and Frans Stiene, *The Reiki Sourcebook,* Winchester, O Books, page 95.

42 "The vajra is regarded as the symbol of highest spiritual power which is irresistible and invincible. It is therefore compared to the diamond, which is capable of cutting asunder any other substance, but which itself cannot be cut by anything." Quoted from *Foundations of Tibetan Mysticism,* Eastford, Martino Publishing, by Lama Govinda, page 61.

43 Steve Gooch, *Buddho-EnerSense Level 2 manual,* 2014.

44 Questions have been raised over whether the Master Symbol (Symbol 4) is a Reiki symbol at all. Reiki Master, Hiroshi Doi confirmed its authenticity when he said that an Aikido Shihan, whose grandfather had trained with Usui, informed him that Usui used to show Symbol 4 to his Shinpiden students (Frans Stiene's *Reiki Insights,* Winchester, Ayni Books, page 134). If you wish to explore this topic it would be worthwhile reading William Rand's piece, *Origin of the Usui Reiki Master Symbol* in *An Evidence Based History of Reiki,* Southfield, International Centre for Reiki Training, pages 82–85 followed by James Deacon's commentary on the subject; *The Reiki Symbol That (Supposedly) Never Was...* on his *Reiki Pages* here: *http://www.aetw.org/reiki_symbolsM2.htm.*

45 Steve Gooch, *Reiki Jin Kei Do: The Way of Compassion & Wisdom,* Winchester, O Books, pages 38–41.

46 Don Beckett, *Reiki, the True Story,* Berkeley, Frog Books, page 155.

47 Steve Gooch, *Reiki Jin Kei Do Level 3 manual,* 2012.

48 Shakyamuni is the historical Buddha that lived roughly 2600 years ago. His name was Siddhartha Gautama, whilst "Shakyamuni" relates to the Shakya clan from which he came.

Vessantara, *Meeting the Buddhas: A Guide to Buddhas, Bodhisattvas, and Tantric Deities,* Birmingham, Windhorse Publications, page 316.

50 Bronwen and Frans Stiene, *The Japanese Art of Reiki,* Ripley, O Books, page 123.

51 Gordon and Dorothy Bell, *Reiki Jin Kei Do Level 2 manual,* 1996.

52 Rob Preece, *The Psychology of Buddhist Tantra,* Ithaca, Snow Lion, page 68.

Chapter 4

1 The use of *chakras* in Reiki has in recent years been dismissed as being an importation from Western New Age thought and nothing to do with the original system. Although this is probably true, *chakras* do in fact have a significant role to play in the practice of Reiki. It should be understood, however, that we are talking here about the tantric (esoteric) Buddhist conception of *chakras* and not the Hindu understanding of them. Lama Govinda: "The Hindu system emphasizes more the static side of the centers and their connexions with elementary nature, by identifying them with the fundamental forces of the universe.... The Buddhist system is less concerned with the static-objective side of the chakras, but rather with that which flows through them, with their dynamic functions, i.e., with the transformation of that current of cosmic or nature-energies into spiritual potentialities." This understanding of the way the *chakra* system works from a Buddhist standpoint, is exactly in line with that promoted by many who work with them in the Reiki community. It is often claimed that as Usui, the founder of Reiki was Japanese, that he would default to working with the *tanden* system (which would seem to be the case) and would not have used the *chakra* system. It is worth noting that, according to Frank Petter (*This Is Reiki,*

Twin Lakes, Lotus Press, page 165) and Jojan Jonker *(Reiki: The Transmigration of a Japanese Spiritual Healing System,* Zurich, Lit Verlag, page 141) Usui was a follower of Jodo Shinshu Buddhism (a branch of Pure Land Buddhism); he is in fact buried at a Pure Land (Shin) Buddhist temple. Others, such as Frans Stiene have claimed he was Tendai (*The Reiki Sourcebook,* Winchester, O Books, pages 56 and 98). Whether a follower or not, he was almost certainly very familiar with Tendai (and possibly Shingon) Buddhism and therefore well versed in the practices of Mikkyo (of which Tendai/Shingon is an expression). Mikkyo is a school of esoteric Buddhism and was influenced by Shintoism and later by Chinese Esoteric Buddhism, Onmyōdō, Taoism and later still, Tibetan Buddhism. It cannot therefore be dismissed that Usui might have referenced and worked with the *chakra* system on some level, as it was probably an innate part of his understanding of the way energy works within the subtle body of the human being.

2 Interestingly, energy concentration points that correspond directly with the four uppermost *chakras* (called *seishin shuchu ichi* in Japanese) are worked upon energetically in Tendai and Shingon Buddhism and suggest an affinity with the concept of Reiki attunements/*reiju*.

3 A useful way of looking at the correspondence between the *tanden* system and the *chakra* system was put forward in a discussion called *Compare Dan Tien to Chakra?* on The Dao Bums website (*https://www.thedaobums.com/topic/6876-compare-dan-tien-to-chakra/*), where it was suggested that if you were to draw three circles, joined at their circumference, these would represent the three *tandens* (or *dan tien* in Chinese). Then put a dot in the middle of each circle, which represents the three elixir fields (earth, heart, heaven), then drew a line through the circles so that it passed through the dots, you would have seven distinct points which

correspond to the *chakra* system, with the three elixir fields corresponding directly to the Sacral, Heart and Third Eye *chakras*.

4 Bronwen and Frans Stiene quote Morihei Ueshiba, the founder of Aikido in relation to this point: "Sensei, why is it that when I practice with you in the dôjô my work is so smooth, yet when I practice at home alone, I can never achieve these same heights of excellence?" Ueshiba replied, "Because in this dôjô you are One with me and I am One with you." (*https://ihreiki.com/blog/everything_about_reiju/*).

5 *Nadi* literally means "stream" and there are thought to be hundreds of thousands of these subtle energy streams within the body.

6 From an esoteric Buddhist psychological perspective, we can say that direct experience of the energy in Reiki starts as an immediate intuition of reality called *Jnana* (which exists outside of our concept of time) that transcends our normal concepts of subject and object. This primal faculty knows a phenomenon before the mind/intellect makes judgments and forms opinions and labels it. It is being perceived on a level that precedes the mind's ability to structure the raw sense data. The mind calls upon previous experiences and other sense data to structure the phenomena, so this is why we have a concept of Reiki energy in flow or manifesting through various energy centers. It is entirely down to the functioning of the mind that our experience of Reiki is organized in such a way to conform with the expected experience, as this draws on sensory data that are common to everyone. The world and our experience of it, is created by the mind, but *Jnana* is prior to the mind and so is beyond the mind. The experience of Reiki flow therefore is a direct *Jnana-ic* perception that is then constructed by the mind to conform to the given experiences of Reiki practitioners.

7 The term "elixir field" is one that is common within

Chinese Taoism as well as within Japanese concepts of energy. As Daniel Reid has pointed out in his classic work *Chi Gung: Harnessing the Power of the Universe,* (London, Simon & Schuster) the lower elixir field, which is just below the navel and associated with the sexual organs is where primordial essence (*jing*) resides. The middle elixir field is focused on the solar plexus and the adrenal glands is where primordial energy (*chi*) is located, and the upper elixir field in the center of the head and associated with the pituitary and pineal glands, is where primordial spirit (*shen*) resides. In Japanese, *jing* is translated as *sei, chi* as *ki* and *shen* is translated as *shin*.

8 Samsen, J. and Hanson, H. (n.d.). *The Dan Tien — Three Major Energy Megalopolises of the Body*. The Gathering – Metaphysical Guidebook: *https://metaphysicalguidebook.wordpress.com/3-2/the-dan-tien-three-major-energy-megalopolises-of-the-body/*

9 Hansen-Buth, B. (2007). *Traditional Reiki Energy System – the Hara*. Reiki Artist Studio ~ Reiki Classes, Services & Gifts: *http://www.reikiartist.com/2007/12/traditional-reiki-energy-system-the-hara/*

10 This is a call to take up the practice of Abdominal Breathing – a technique for building energy and then using it for cleansing energy pathways and balancing the opposing forces of *yin* and *yang* (*in* and *yo* in Japanese).

11 The New Yoga. (n.d.). *TANTRA AND TAOISM On their Essential Nature and Relation*: *http://www.thenewyoga.org/tantra_and_taoism.htm*

12 Daniel Reid gives an excellent description of the Three Treasures and how they relate to wider aspects of what it is to be a human being in Chapter 4 of *Chi Gung: Harnessing the Power of the Universe* (London, Simon & Schuster).

13 Quoted in *Shingon Esoteric Buddhism: A Handbook for Followers,* Fresno, Shingon Buddhist International Institute,

by Yusei Arai.

14 Frans Stiene discusses the nature of The Three Treasures in relation to Reiki on page 29 of *The Inner Heart of Reiki*, Winchester, Ayni Books. This whole chapter is an excellent discussion of The Three Treasures and their place in the system of Reiki.

15 Author Torsten A. Lange describes the practice of *Koki-Ho* on page 108 of *Reiki: Heal your Body and your Life with the Power of Universal Energy,* (London, Hay House): 1. Connect to Reiki. 2. Take a deep breath and bring your lips together. 3. Draw the power symbol with your tongue (ed. you can just visualise the symbol – no need to draw it with the tongue), and keep the tongue pressed against the back of the teeth. 4. Breathe this energy out to the affected area of the person's body. If you don't have the power symbol to work with, you can just leave that step out and do it without the symbol.

16 Quoted by Frans Stiene in *The Inner Heart of Reiki: Rediscovering Your True Self,* Winchester, Ayni Books, page 30 and taken from the *Dainichi-kyo Sutra.*

17 The Japanese meditation and energy awareness methods such as *Joshin Kokyu Ho, Seishin Toitsu* and *Kenyoku Ho* first started to appear in the West due to the research of German Reiki Master and author Frank Arjava Petter (*The Original Reiki Handbook of Dr Mikao Usui,* Twin Lakes, Lotus Press) and were brought to further prominence by Hiroshi Doi (*Iyashino Gendai Reiki-ho: Modern Reiki Method for Healing,* Coquitlam, Fraser Journal Publishing) and later Bronwen and Frans Stiene in their book *The Japanese Art of Reiki,* Ropley, O Books.

18 *Reiki Jin Kei Do* is a lineage of Reiki coming from the Buddhist monk and tantric master Seiji Takamori, that was transmitted to Ranga Premaratna in the early 1990s. It contains teachings and practices related to the origins

of Usui's Reiki that are not contained in other traditions of Reiki, most specifically, the *Buddho* meditation, which is thought to be the meditation that Mikao Usui practiced on Mt Kurama when he had his enlightenment experience – a significant and extensively reported moment in the development of the Reiki system. See my book; *Reiki Jin Kei Do: The Way of Compassion & Wisdom* (Winchester, O Books) for further information.

19 This practice is not to be confused with the Forest Monks' practice of chanting *Buddho* to help instil one-pointed concentration.

20 Christopher Markert, (1998) *Dan Tien: Your Secret Energy Center,* York Beach, Samuel Weiser, Inc., page 93.

21 Quoted on the excellent blog of Mike Garofalo called *Cloud Hands*, which you can find here: *http://mpgtaijiquan.blogspot.com/2017/03/tao-te-ching-chapter-10.html*.

22 Daniel Reid writes eloquently about the art and science of breathing and the functions and benefits of diaphragmic breathing on page 128 of *Chi-Gung: Harnessing the Power of the Universe* (London, Simon & Schuster).

23 *Dhyana* (or *jhana* in Pali) is the word that the Japanese later pronounced as *Zen*.

Chapter 5

1 Sadhguru is an Indian, mystic, yogi and author who founded the *Isha Foundation* in 1992: a non-profit spiritual organisation that offers yoga programs around the world. It is also involved in various social outreach, educational and environmental initiatives.

2 Sadhguru's video relating to the practice of Reiki is fundamentally flawed (*Sadhguru Why One Should not do Reiki to Avoid Karma*), not because of what Sadhguru has to say, but because of the beliefs and assumptions made in the statement that was put to him: "If you give Reiki to

somebody you are actually taking on their karmic patterns." This is of course, nonsense and has no relationship to the system of Reiki. Sadhguru's responses were framed around this statement and addressed it as if it were true. Sadhguru's words were presented in a YouTube video that has now been deleted. You can find some similar reflections from Sadhguru on the practice of Reiki here: *https://www.youtube.com/watch?v=8B85d8h9kFU.*

3 *Why do you tell people not to do healing? Sadhguru*. This was a YouTube video that has now been deleted. You can find some similar reflections from Sadhguru on the practice of Reiki here: *https://www.youtube.com/watch?v=8B85d8h9kFU.*

4 Bodo Baginski and Shalila Sharamon, *Reiki Universal Energy,* Mendocino, LifeRhythm, page 107. This is one of the early books on Reiki published in the West and a real classic of its time.

5 *The Online Etymology Dictionary*: *https://www.etymonline.com/search?q=heal*

6 The microcosmic orbit is a Taoist Qigong energy cultivation practice, involving deep breathing in conjunction with meditation and concentration techniques.

7 Liang, S. & Wu, W, *Qigong Empowerment: A Guide to Medical, Taoist, Buddhist, Wushu Energy Cultivation*, Rhode Island, The Way of the Dragon Publishing, page 227–228.

8 Frank Arjava Petter, *This Is Reiki,* Twin Lakes, Lotus Press, page 201.

9 Referenced in the article *Buddhism and Healing* by Professor Alfred Bloom on Shin Dharma Net at: *http://bschawaii.org/shindharmanet/healing/*

10 Frank Arjava Petter, *This Is Reiki,* Twin Lakes, Lotus Press, page 202.

11 See my book *Reiki Jin Kei Do: The Way of Compassion and Wisdom,* Winchester, O Books, page 128–130 for a fuller explanation of this meditation practice.

12 See *Chi Gung: Harnessing the Power of the Universe,* London, Simon & Schuster, pages 58 60 by Daniel Reid for a fuller explanation of the effects different postures have on energy flow.

Chapter 6

1 The Four Noble Truths, along with the Eightfold Path are the essence of the whole of Buddhist teaching, and were originally expounded by the Buddha more than 2500 years ago.

2 See *https://en.wikipedia.org/wiki/Dhammacakkappavattana Sutta*

3 See *https://www.accesstoinsight.org/tipitaka/dn/dn.16.1-6.vaji.html*

4 Fischer, N. (2017). *Suffering Opens the Real Path* can be found at *www.lionsroar.com/the-real-path/*

5 See *http://bschawaii.org/shindharmanet/healing/*

6 Williams, M., Teasdale, J., Segal, Z., and Kabat-Zinn, J. (2007). *The Mindful Way through Depression*, New York, The Guilford Press, page 32.

7 The concept of the negativity bias has been extensively discussed by Dr Rick Hanson. For information about his work, see *https://www.rickhanson.net/the-science-of-positive-brain-change/* Information relating specifically to the negativity bias can be found in *Negative Information Weighs More Heavily on the Brain: The Negativity Bias in Evaluative Categorizations*, a copy of which can be found here: *https://media.rickhanson.net/KeyScientificPapers/Negativity_Bias_in_Judgments.pdf*

8 Burch, V., and Penman, D. (2013). *Mindfulness for Health,* London, Piatkus, pages 157–158.

9 Quoted in Burch, V., and Penman, D. (2013). *Mindfulness for Health*. London: Piatkus. Page 159 from Hanson, R. (2009). *Buddha's Brain: The Practical Neuroscience of Happiness, Love*

and Wisdom, Oakland, New Harbinger Publications.

10 Moore, C. (2019). *What Is the Negativity Bias and How Can It Be Overcome?* Available at: *https://positivepsychology.com/3-steps-negativity-bias/*

11 Preece, R. (2006). *The Psychology of Buddhist Tantra,* Ithaca, Snow Lion, page 61.

12 Williams, M., Teasdale, J., Segal, Z. and Kabat-Zinn, J. (2007). *The Mindful Way through Depression*, New York, The Guilford Press, page 162.

13 Quoted in Baker. I. (1997). *The Tibetan Art of Healing*, London, Thames & Hudson, page 69.

14 Nairn, R., Choden, Regan-Addis, H. (2019). *From Mindfulness to Insight*, Boulder, Shambhala Publications, pages 85–86.

15 Williams, M., Teasdale, J., Segal, Z. and Kabat-Zinn, J. (2007). *The Mindful Way through Depression*, New York, The Guilford Press, page 128.

16 Burch, V., and Penman, D. (2013). *Mindfulness for Health*, London, Piatkus, page 21.

17 Zeidan, F., Emerson, N., Farris, S., Ray, J., Jung, Y., McHaffie, J., & Coghill, R. (2015). Mindfulness Meditation-Based Pain Relief Employs Different Neural Mechanisms Than Placebo and Sham Mindfulness Meditation-Induced Analgesia. *Journal of Neuroscience*, 35(46), 15307-15325.

18 Burch, V., and Penman, D. (2013). *Mindfulness for Health*, London, Piatkus, page 24.

19 Kuyken, W., Hayes, R., Barrett, B., Byng, R., Dalgleish, T. and Kessler, D. et al. (2015). *Effectiveness and cost-effectiveness of mindfulness-based cognitive therapy compared with maintenance antidepressant treatment in the prevention of depressive relapse or recurrence (PREVENT): a randomised controlled trial, The Lancet*, 386, pages 63–73. *https://www.thelancet.com/journals/lancet/article/PIIS0140-6736(14)62222-4/fulltext*

20 Burch, V. (2008) *Living Well with Pain and Illness*, London, Piatkus, page 29.

21 This topic was discussed at length on the *Dhamma Wheel* Buddhist forum. You can find the text from the Arrow Sutra here: *https://dhammawheel.com/viewtopic.php?t=13429#p199822*

22 Skinner, J. D., and Bladen, S. (2018). *Practical Zen for Health Wealth and Mindfulness*, London, Singing Dragon, pages 48–49.

23 Statistic quoted in Skinner, J. D., and Bladen, S. (2018). *Practical Zen for Health Wealth and Mindfulness*, London, Singing Dragon, pages 47.

24 Williams, M., Teasdale, J., Segal, Z., and Kabat-Zinn, J. (2007). *The Mindful Way through Depression*, New York, The Guilford Press, pages 100–101.

25 Skinner, J. D., and Bladen, S. (2018). *Practical Zen for Health Wealth and Mindfulness*, London, Singing Dragon, pages 57–62.

26 For a good description of the RAIN approach, see Nairn, R., Choden, and Regan-Addis, H. (2019), *From Mindfulness to Insight* (Boulder, Shambhala Publications). You could also check out Tara Brach's book, *Radical Compassion* (London, Rider), which I feel is a more compassion-loaded version of essentially the same process.

27 The classic version of RAIN ascribes "Non-identification" to the letter N, however, as Tara Brach, I think quite rightly, points out, non-identification is actually something that is impossible to "do," unlike Recognising, Allowing and Investigating. Awareness of non-identification arises unbidden through the practice. Brach has therefore relabeled "N" as meaning "Nurturing" which seems to me an eminently better "doing" label, that in combination with the others gives way to the "being2" of Non-identification. See Brach, T. (2020) *Radical Compassion*. London, Rider.

Chapter 7

1 Sandy C. Newbigging, *3 Steps to Harness the Power of Om to Transform Your Life*, available here: *https://www.*

mindbodygreen.com/0-5132/3-Steps-to-Harness-the-Power-of-Om-to-Transform-Your-Life.html

2 Simon Heather, *Om – The Primordial Sound,* available here: *http://www.simonheather.co.uk/pages/articles/aum.pdf*

3 You can find a full translation of this *Upanishad* here: *https://archive.org/details/maitriormaitrya00cowegoog/page/n13*

4 Vessantara, *Meeting the Buddhas: A Guide to Buddhas, Bodhisattvas, and Tantric Deities,* Birmingham, Windhorse Publications, page 124.

5 Vessantara, *Meeting the Buddhas: A Guide to Buddhas, Bodhisattvas, and Tantric Deities,* Birmingham, Windhorse Publications, page 125.

6 Sangharakshita, *Living with Kindness: The Buddha's Teachings on Metta,* Cambridge, Windhorse Publications, page 3.

7 Lee Kane, *Scientific Buddhist: Peer Reviewed Studies Demonstrate Buddhist Metta Loving Kindness Meditation Can Slow Aging, Increase Brain Matter, and Decrease PTSD and Schizophrenia – Ten Benefits of Compassion* in *Buddha Weekly* at: *https://buddhaweekly.com/scientific-buddhist-peer-reviewed-studies-demonstrate-buddhist-metta-loving-kindness-meditation-can-slow-aging-increase-brain-matter-decrease-ptsd-schizophrenia-ten-benefits-com/*

8 *The Dhammapada* is a collection of the sayings of the Buddha.

9 Bhante Gunaratana, *Loving Kindness in Plain English,* Somerville, Wisdom Publications, page 1.

10 Sharon Salzberg, *Loving Kindness: The Revolutionary Art of Happiness*, Boulder, Shambhala Publications Inc., page 19.

11 Sangharakshita, *Living with Kindness: The Buddha's Teachings on Metta,* Cambridge, Windhorse Publications, page 14.

12 Sangharakshita, *Living with Kindness: The Buddha's Teachings on Metta,* Cambridge, Windhorse Publications, pages15–16.

13 Acharya Buddharakkhita, *Metta: The Philosophy and Practice of Universal Love* available here: *https://accesstoinsight.org/lib/authors/buddharakkhita/wheel365.html*

14 Sangharashita, *Living with Kindness: The Buddha's Teachings on Metta,* Cambridge, Windhorse Publications, page 104.

15 From an internet meme which you can find here: *https://twitter.com/OmAhHum2019/status/1183653335406206977/photo/1*

16 As reported in the article *18 Science-Based Reasons to Try Loving-Kindness Meditation Today!* by Emmamseppala, which can be found here: *https://emmaseppala.com/18-science-based-reasons-try-loving-kindness-meditation-today/*

17 Bodhipaksa, *The Science of Lovingkindness*: *https://www.wildmind.org/blogs/on-practice/the-science-of-lovingkindness*

18 Emmamseppala, *18 Science-Based Reasons to Try Loving-Kindness Meditation Today!*: *https://emmaseppala.com/18-science-based-reasons-try-loving-kindness-meditation-today/*

19 Emmamseppala, *18 Science-Based Reasons to Try Loving-Kindness Meditation Today!*: *https://emmaseppala.com/18-science-based-reasons-try-loving-kindness-meditation-today/*

20 Tai Bendit-Shtull, *Combating Implicit Bias with Meditation*: *https://repository.upenn.edu/cgi/viewcontent.cgi?article=1149&context=wharton_research_scholars*

21 Bodhipaksa, *The Science of Lovingkindness*: *https://www.wildmind.org/blogs/on-practice/the-science-of-lovingkindness*

22 Jack Kornfield, *A Path with Heart*, London, Rider, page 19.

23 Sharon Salzberg, *Loving-Kindness: The Revolutionary Art of Happiness*, Boulder, Shambhala Publications In., page 46.

Chapter 8

1 Quoted in *The Tibetan Art of Healing* by Ian Baker, London, Thames & Hudson, page 164.

2 Ian Baker, *The Tibetan Art of Healing,* London, Thames & Hudson, page 170.

3 Robert Fueston, *Reiki Transmission of Light Vol 1,* New Delhi, New Age Books, page 117.

4 Robert Fueston, *Reiki Transmission of Light Vol 1,* New Delhi,

New Age Books, page 117.

5 Robert Fueston, *Reiki Transmission of Light Vol 1*, New Delhi, New Age Books, page 120.

6 Many of the early books on the system of Reiki report that Usui traveled to China where he learnt Chinese and then went on to northern India, prior to his return to Japan.

7 Master Shou-Yu Liang & Wen-Ching Wu, *Qigong Empowerment: A Guide to Medical, Taoist, Buddhist Wushu Energy Cultivation*, Rhode Island, The Way of the Dragon Publishing, page 137 and 145–146.

8 It's worth noting that the Buddho meditation, taught within the tradition of Reiki Jin Kei Do which requires a series of empowerments, has a direct relationship to the *Bodhisattva* Avalokiteshvara which in turn relates directly to an allied esoteric Buddhist Qigong practice called *Chi Nadi*. These two components have a powerful symbiotic relationship and are considered within the tradition to have a direct causal relationship to the origins of secular Reiki. See my book *Reiki Jin Kei Do: The Way of Compassion & Wisdom*, Winchester, O Books, page 97 for further information.

9 Kenneth S. Connor, *The Way of Qigong*, New York, Ballantine Books, page 45.

10 The great tantric master, Padmasambhava when asked by the Dakini Yeshe Tsogyal about the necessity for tantric empowerments said: "To exert yourself in study and so forth without attending a master and without having received the empowerments, you will have no result and your efforts will be wasted. Empowerment is the entrance to the Secret Mantra. To enter the Secret Mantra without the empowerments being conferred is pointless, since it will yield no result and your stream of being will be ruined" (From: *Padmasambhava Guru Rinpoche, Dakini Teachings*, page 60. Rangjung Yeshe Publications. Kindle Edition).

11 Preece, R. (2006). *The Psychology of Buddhist Tantra*, Ithaca,

Snow Lion, page 81.

12 *Shen* can be described as spirit and relates to the mind. It could be called consciousness or the quality of mental vitality. There are many variations on the definition of *shen* within the context of Qigong and Traditional Chinese Medicine. See *https://www.sacredlotus.com/go/foundations-chinese-medicine/get/shen-spirit-chinese-medicine* for a good description of *shen* and how it fits into the concepts of Traditional Chinese Medicine.

13 Jwing-Ming, Yang, Dr (2003). *Qigong Meditation Embryonic Breathing*, Boston, YMAA Publication Center, pages 81 and 149.

14 Germer, C. (2009). *The Mindful Path to Self-Compassion,* New York, The Guilford Press, page 97.

15 The *skandhas* are the physical matter that makes up our bodies, our emotions and feelings that arise from our senses, our thinking and intellectual reasoning, our mental formations such as habits and prejudices and finally consciousness and non-judgmental awareness.

16 HH Dalai Lama, (2008). *How to See Yourself as You Really Are,* London, Rider, page 127.

17 Nāgārjuna. and Garfield, J. (1995). *The Fundamental Wisdom of The Middle Way*, New York, Oxford University Press, page 60.

18 *Shunyata* simply means emptiness. It is sometimes translated as voidness.

19 Kushner, L. Rabbi. (2006). *Kabbalah: A Love Story,* New York, Broadway Books, page124.

20 Williams, M., Teasdale, J., Segal, Z. & Kabat-Zinn, J. (2007). *The Mindful Way Through Depression,* New York, The Guilford Press, page 226.

21 Kabat-Zinn, J. (2019). *A Meditation for Resting in Awareness.* [online] Mindful. Available at: *https://www.mindful.org/a-meditation-for-resting-in-awareness/* [Accessed 9 June 2020].

22 Nairn, R., Choden, Regan-Addis, H., (2019). *From Mindfulness to Insight*, Boulder, Shambhala Publications Inc., page 264–265.

Chapter 9

1 Germer, C. (2009). *The Mindful Path to Self-Compassion*, New York, The Guilford Press, page 229.

2 The Three Minute Breathing Space was developed by cognitive therapists, Zindel Segal, John Teasdale and Mark Williams as a part of their MBCT (Mindfulness Based Cognitive Therapy) program. A good little article by Zindel Segal about the reasons why this practice was developed was published in *Mindful* magazine and can be accessed here: *https://www.mindful.org/the-three-minute-breathing-space-practice/*

3 Williams, M.,Teasdale, J., Segal, Z. and Kabat-Zinn, J. (2009) *The Mindful Way through Depression*, New York, The Guilford Press, page 190.

4 Breathworks is one of the world's lead bodies for research and training in the area of the medical and health benefits of mindfulness meditation. You can find out more about the Breathworks approach to mindfulness at *https://www.breathworks-mindfulness.org.uk/*

Afterword

1 Nairn, R., Choden, Regan-Addis, R. (2019). *From Mindfulness to Insight*, Boulder, Shambhala Publications Inc., pages 266–280, gives an excellent description of this practice.

Bibliography

An Evidence Based History of Reiki. (2015). Southfield: International Center for Reiki Training.

Arai, Y. (1997). *Shingon Esoteric Buddhism: A Handbook for Followers.* Fresno: Shingon Buddhist International Institute.

Asai Shotokan Association International. (n.d.). *What Is Tanden?* [online] Available at: http://asaikarate.com/what-is-tanden-%E4%B8%B9%E7%94%B0%E3%81%A8%E3%81%AF%E4%BD%95%E3%81%9E%E3%82%84%EF%BC%9F/ [Accessed 8 Apr. 2019].

Ashley-Farrand, T. (1999). *Healing Mantras.* New York: Ballantine Wellspring.

Baginski, B. and Sharamon, S. (1988). *Reiki Universal Energy.* Mendocino: LifeRhythm.

Baker, I. (1997). *The Tibetan Art of Healing.* London: Thames & Hudson.

Beckett, D. (2009). *Reiki, the True Story.* Berkeley: Frog Books.

Bell, G. (1998). *Healing in Buddhism.* [online] Healing Touch. Available at: http://www.healing-touch.co.uk/pa-medb.htm [Accessed 9 Jun. 2019].

Bendit-Shtull, T. (2017). *Combating Implicit Bias with Meditation.* [ebook] The Wharton School, University of Pennsylvania. Available at: https://repository.upenn.edu/cgi/viewcontent.cgi?article=1149&context=wharton_research_scholars [Accessed 14 Nov. 2019].

Birdfield, T. (2003). *Buddho-EnerSense Level 3 Manual.* Dorset: Tony Birdfield.

Bloom, A. (n.d.). *Buddhism and Healing.* [online] Shin Dharma Net. Available at: http://bschawaii.org/shindharmanet/healing/ [Accessed 7 Aug. 2019].

Boggenpoel, E. (2019). *10-Minute Mindfulness.* Horncastle: Mortons Media Group Ltd.

Bodhipaksa (2011). *The science of lovingkindness – Wildmind.* [online] Wildmind. Available at: https://www.wildmind.org/blogs/on-practice/the-science-of-lovingkindness [Accessed 29 Oct. 2019].

Brach, T. (2020). *Radical Compassion.* London: Rider.

Brady, A. and Waring, R. (n.d.). *What Is a Chakra?* [online] The Yoga People. Available at: http://theyogapeople.com/what-is-a-*chakra*/ [Accessed 4 Apr. 2019].

Brazier, D. (2001). *Zen Therapy: A Buddhist Approach to Psychotherapy.* London: Robinson.

Brecher, P. (1997). *Thorsons Principles of Tai Chi.* London: Thorsons.

Buddharakkhita, A. (1995). *Metta: The Philosophy and Practice of Universal Love.* [online] Accesstoinsight.org. Available at: https://accesstoinsight.org/lib/authors/buddharakkhita/wheel365.html [Accessed 25 Sep. 2019].

Burch. V. (2008). *Living Well with Pain & Illness.* London: Piatkus.

Burch, V. and Penman, D. (2013). *Mindfulness for Health*. London: Piatkus.

Byakko Shinko Kai. (n.d.). *KOTODAMA – The power of words.* [online] Available at: https://byakko.org/philosophy/kotodama-the-power-of-words/ [Accessed 14 Jul. 2019].

Chinabuddhismencyclopedia.com. (2019). *Amitabha – Chinese Buddhist Encyclopedia.* [online] Available at: http://www.chinabuddhismencyclopedia.com/en/index.php?title=Amitabha [Accessed 21 Aug. 2019].

Chinabuddhismencyclopedia.com. (2019). *Wangdu: The Prayer which magnetizes all that appears and all that exists – Chinese Buddhist Encyclopedia.* [online] Available at: http://www.chinabuddhismencyclopedia.com/en/index.php?title=Wangdu:_The_Prayer_which_magnetizes_all_that_appears_and_all_that_exists#The_Meaning_of_the_Words_-_om_ah_hung_hrih [Accessed 21 Aug. 2019].

Chowdhury, M. (2019). *What Is Loving-Kindness Meditation?*

(Incl. 4 Scripts + YouTube Videos). [online] PositivePsychology.com. Available at: https://positivepsychology.com/loving-kindness-meditation/ [Accessed 24 Oct. 2019].

Clifford, T. (1989). *The Diamond Healing: Tibetan Buddhist Medicine and Psychiatry*. Wellingborough: Crucible.

Connor, K. (1997). *The Way of Qigong: The Art and Science of Chinese Energy Healing*. New York: Ballantine Books.

Cowell, E. (1870). *Maitri or Maitrayaniya Upnishad*. London: W.M. Watts.

Deacon, J. (n.d.). *James Deacon's Reiki Pages*. [online] Available at: http://www.aetw.org [Accessed 15th Aug. 2019].

Deacon, J. (2004). *hon sha ze sho nen / HSZSN (also: hon ja ze sho nen)*. [online] Aetw.org. Available at: http://www.aetw.org/reiki_symbolsD.html [Accessed 25 Aug. 2019].

Deacon, J. (2004). *Chokurei /CKR (Cho Ku Rei / Choku Rei)*. [online] Aetw.org. Available at: http://www.aetw.org/reiki_symbolsP.html [Accessed 12 Nov. 2019].

Deacon, J. (2005). *The Reiki Symbols – Ongoing Research*. [ebook] James Deacon. Available at: http://www.aetw.org/reiki_pdf.htm [Accessed 5 Sep. 2019].

Deacon, J. (2008). *The Japanese Reiki Techniques: Level 2*. 1st ed. [ebook] James Deacon. Available at: http://www.aetw.org/reiki_pdf.htm [Accessed 15 Jul. 2019].

Doi, H. (2000). *Iyashi Gendai Reiki-ho: Modern Reiki Method for Healing*. Coquitlam: Fraser Journal Publishing.

Durckheim, K. (2004). *Hara: The Vital Center of Man*. Rochester: Inner Traditions.

Dyer, W. (2005). *You'll See It When You Believe It*. London: Arrow Books.

Editors of Encyclopaedia Britannica (n.d.). *Pāli language*. [online] Encyclopaedia Britannica. Available at: https://www.britannica.com/topic/Pali-language [Accessed 2 Jun. 2019].

Eastcott, M. (1989). *The Silent Path: A Comprehensive Introduction to the Study of Meditation.* London: Rider.

Ellis, R. (2015). *Reiki and the Hara.* [online] Practical Reiki: The Richard Ellis School of Reiki. Available at: http://www.practicalreiki.com/blog/reiki-and-the-hara/ [Accessed 4 Apr. 2019].

Ellyard, L. (2010). *Reiki Meditations for Beginners.* Twin Lakes. Lotus Press.

En.wikipedia.org. (2020). *Dhammacakkappavattana Sutta.* [online] Available at: https://en.wikipedia.org/wiki/Dhammacakkappavattana_Sutta [Accessed 8 Apr. 2020].

Fueston, R. (2017). *Reiki Transmission of Light Vol 1.* New Delhi: New Age Books.

Frazier, K. (2018). *Engaging in the Flow of Reiki through Its Three Pillars.* [online] AuthorKarenFrazier.com. Available at: https://www.authorkarenfrazier.com/blog/engaging-in-the-flow-of-reiki-through-its-three-pillars [Accessed 20 Apr. 2019].

Garofalo, M. (2017). *Tao Te Ching, Chapter 10.* [online] Cloud Hands. Available at: http://mpgtaijiquan.blogspot.com/2017/03/tao-te-ching-chapter-10.html [Accessed 17 Apr. 2019].

Germer, C. (2009). *The Mindful Path to Self-Compassion.* New York: The Guilford Press.

Gooch, S. (2006). *Reiki Jin Kei Do: The Way of Compassion & Wisdom.* 1st ed. Winchester: O Books.

Gooch, S. (2012). *Reiki Level 1 Manual.* Rugby: Steve Gooch.

Gooch, S. (2014). *Buddho-EnerSense Level 1 Manual.* Rugby: Steve Gooch.

Gooch, S. (2014). *Buddho-EnerSense Level 2 Manual.* Rugby: Steve Gooch.

Gooch, S. (2019). *Why You Should be Wary of Energy Healing.* [Blog] *Steve Gooch: Author, freelance writer, artist.* Available at: https://stevegoochwrites.wordpress.com/2019/03/17/why-you-should-be-wary-of-energy-healing/ [Accessed 3 Apr.

2019].

Govinda, A. (2012). *Foundations of Tibetan Mysticism.* Eastford: Martino Publishing.

Gunaratana, B. (2017). *Longing Kindness in Plain English: The Practice of Metta.* Somerville: Wisdom Publications.

HH Dalai Lama, (5th). (n.d.). *A Practice of Consciousness Transference Involving Amitabha.* [ebook] Available at: https://static.squarespace.com/static/50be4fefe4b0c82b6072c4ed/t/53691321e4b0b561109cff5a/1399395105551/amitabha.pdf [Accessed 24 Aug. 2019].

HH Dalai Lama, and Cutler, H. (1998). *The Art of Happiness: A Handbook for Living*. 1st ed. London: Hodder & Stoughton.

HH Dalai Lama, (2008). *How to See Yourself as You Truly Are.* London: Rider.

Halliwell, E. (2015). *Mindfulness: How to Live Well by Paying Attention.* London: Hay House UK Ltd.

Hanh, T.N. (2013). *Peace of Mind: Becoming Fully Present*. London: Bantam Press.

Hansen-Buth, B. (2007). *Traditional Reiki Energy System – the Hara*. [online] Reiki Artist Studio ~ Reiki Classes, Services & Gifts. Available at: http://www.reikiartist.com/2007/12/traditional-reiki-energy-system-the-hara/ [Accessed 29 Mar. 2019].

Heather, S. (n.d.). *Om – The Primordial Sound*. [ebook] Simon Heather. Available at: http://www.simonheather.co.uk/pages/articles/aum.pdf [Accessed 22 Sep. 2019].

Hennessey, G. (2016). *The Little Mindfulness Workbook.* Bath: Crimson Publishing Ltd.

Holzel, B. and Ott, U. (2007). *Relationships Between Meditation Depth, Absorption, Meditation Practice, and Mindfulness: A Latent Variable Approach.* [ebook] The Journal of Transpersonal Psychology. Available at: http://www.atpweb.org/jtparchive/trps-38-02-179.pdf [Accessed 27 May 2019].

Hosak, M. and Lubeck, W. (2006). *The Big Book of Reiki Symbols.*

Twin Lakes: Lotus Press.

Hotatsumatsue. (2001). *Hotsuma-Tsutae.* [online] Available at: http://hotsuma.gr.jp/futomani-e.html [Accessed 18 Aug. 2019].

Ito, T., Larsen, J., Smith, N., & Cacioppo, J. (1998). *Negative Information Weighs More Heavily on the Brain: The Negativity Bias in Evaluative Categorizations* [ebook]. The American Psychological Association, Inc. Available at: https://media.rickhanson.net/KeyScientificPapers/Negativity_Bias_in_Judgments.pdf [Accessed 8 Apr. 2020].

Johari, H. (1986). *Tools for Tantra.* Vermont: Destiny Books.

Jonker, J. (2016). *Reiki: The Transmigration of a Japanese Spiritual Healing Practice (Nijmegen Buddhist and Asian Studies).* Zurich: Lit Verlag.

Jwing-Ming, Yang, Dr (2003). *Qigong Meditation Embryonic Breathing.* Boston: YMAA Publication Center.

Kabat-Zinn, J. (2019). *A Meditation for Resting in Awareness.* [online] Mindful. Available at: https://www.mindful.org/a-meditation-for-resting-in-awareness/ [Accessed 9 June 2020].

Kane, L. (2019). *The Better Way: Standing Meditation? For those with injuries, arthritis or a sleepy mind, standing can help us achieve mindfulness.* [online] Buddha Weekly. Available at: https://buddhaweekly.com/the-better-way-standing-meditation/ [Accessed 31 Jul. 2019].

Kane, L. (2019). *Scientific Buddhist: Peer Reviewed Studies Demonstrate Buddhist Metta Loving Kindness Meditation Can Slow Aging, Increase Brain Matter, and Decrease PTSD and Schizophrenia – Ten Benefits of Compassion.* [online] Buddha Weekly. Available at: https://buddhaweekly.com/scientific-buddhist-peer-reviewed-studies-demonstrate-buddhist-*metta*-loving-kindness-meditation-can-slow-aging-increase-brain-matter-decrease-ptsd-schizophrenia-ten-benefits-com/ [Accessed 31 Jul. 2019].

Kawagoe, A. (2013). *Taka-ma-HARA, or High HARA – the celestial shining mountain peak; the Japanese elixir field; the navel-belly of the earth finds cognates elsewhere (Comparative etymology).* [online] Heritage of Japan. Available at: https://heritageofjapan.wordpress.com/2013/11/05/taka-ma-hara-or-high-hara-the-celestial-shining-mountain-peak-the-japanese-elixir-field-the-navel-belly-of-the-earth-finds-cognates-elsewhere-comparative-etymology/ [Accessed 8 Apr. 2019].

Kelly, M. (2000). *Reiki and the Healing Buddha.* Twin Lakes: Lotus Press.

Khanna, M. (2003). *Yantra: The Tantric Symbol of Cosmic Unity.* London: Thames & Hudson.

Khema, A. (1991). *When the Iron Eagle Flies: Buddhism for the West*. London: Arkana.

Khema, A. (1997). *Who Is Myself? A Guide to Buddhist Meditation.* Somerville: Wisdom Publications.

King, T. (n.d.). *Attunements and Empowerments: What Is the Difference?* [online] Reiki Evolution. Available at: https://www.reiki-evolution.co.uk/attunements-and-empowerments-what-is-the-difference/ [Accessed 1 Apr. 2019].

King, T. (n.d.). *Mindfulness and Compassion in Reiki Healing.* [online] Reiki Evolution. Available at: https://www.reiki-evolution.co.uk/mindfulness-and-compassion/ [Accessed 28 May 2019].

King, T. (2001). *Japanese Reiki Techniques Course.* Braintree: Reiki Evolution.

Kleine, C. (n.d.). *Buddhist Monks as Healers in Early and Medieval Japan*. [ebook] Christoph Kleine. Available at: https://www.researchgate.net/publication/284187272_Buddhist_Monks_as_Healers_in_Early_and_Medieval_Japan [Accessed 21 Aug. 2019].

Kornfield, J. (1994). *A Path with Heart.* London: Rider.

Kushner, L. Rabbi. (2006). *Kabbalah: A Love Story*. New York: Broadway Books.

Kuyken, W., Hayes, R., Barrett, B., Byng, R., Dalgleish, T. and Kessler, D. et al., (2015). *Effectiveness and cost-effectiveness of mindfulness-based cognitive therapy compared with maintenance antidepressant treatment in the prevention of depressive relapse or recurrence (PREVENT): a randomised controlled trial, The Lancet*, 386, pages 63–73. Available at: *https://www.thelancet.com/journals/lancet/article/PIIS0140-6736(14)62222-4/fulltext* [Accessed 30 Apr. 2020].

Kyabgon, T. (2015). *Karma: What It Is, What It Isn't, Why It Matters.* Boston: Shambhala.

Lange, T. (2015). *Reiki: Heal Your Body and Your Life with the Power of Universal Energy.* London: Hay House UK Ltd.

Liang, S. and Wu, W. (1997). *Qigong Empowerment: A Guide to Medical, Taoist, Buddhist, Wushu Energy Cultivation*. 1st ed. Rhode Island: The Way of the Dragon Publishing.

Lion's Roar. (2016). *What Are the Three Kayas?* [online] Available at: https://www.lionsroar.com/buddhism-by-the-numbers-the-three-kayas/ [Accessed 6 Sep. 2019].

Lubeck, W., Petter, F. and Rand, W. (2001). *The Spirit of Reiki: The Complete Handbook of the Reiki System*. 1st ed. Twin Lakes: Lotus Press / Shangri-La.

Markert, C. (1998). *Dan Tien: Your Secret Energy Center.* York Beach: Samuel Weiser, Inc.

Miller, A. (1982). *Japan's Modern Myth: The Language and Beyond.* New York & Tokyo: John Weatherhill.

Mindful: Healthy Mind, Healthy Life. (2014). *What Is Mindfulness?* [online] Available at: https://www.mindful.org/what-is-mindfulness/ [Accessed 25 Apr. 2019].

Moore, C. (2019). *What Is the Negativity Bias and How Can It Be Overcome?* [online] Available at: https://positivepsychology.com/3-steps-negativity-bias/ [Accessed 30 Mar. 2020].

Nāgārjuna. and Garfield, J. (1995). *The Fundamental Wisdom of The Middle Way*. New York: Oxford University Press.

Nairn, R., Choden, Regan-Addis, H. (2019). *From Mindfulness to*

Insight. Boulder: Shambhala Publications Inc.

Nanoo, R. (2015). *Reiki Sutras: Healing Art of the Enlightened.* Rajesh Nanoo.

Nammour, M. 2010). *The World's Energy Within Your Hands.* Beirut: Ciel A Book Company.

Newbigging, S. (2012). *3 Steps to Harness the Power of Om to Transform Your Life*. [online] mindbodygreen. Available at: https://www.mindbodygreen.com/0-5132/3-Steps-to-Harness-the-Power-of-Om-to-Transform-Your-Life.html [Accessed 22 Sep. 2019].

NewBuddhist. (2012). *Dharmakaya, Sambhogakaya, Nirmanakaya*. [online] Available at: https://newbuddhist.com/discussion/13951/Dharmakaya-Sambhogakaya-Nirmanakaya [Accessed 24 Aug. 2019].

NHS. (2018). *Mindfulness*. [online] Available at: https://www.nhs.uk/conditions/stress-anxiety-depression/mindfulness/# [Accessed 25 Apr. 2019].

Nishina, M. (2017). *Reiki and Japan: A Cultural View of Western and Japanese Reiki.* Masaki Nishina.

O'Brien, B. (2019). *What Does "Nirmanakaya" Mean?* [online] Learn Religions. Available at: https://www.learnreligions.com/Nirmanakaya-449847 [Accessed 6 Sep. 2019].

Parrott-Sheffer, C. (n.d.). *Stupa | Buddhism*. [online] Encyclopedia Britannica. Available at: https://www.britannica.com/topic/stupa [Accessed 25 Aug. 2019].

Pearson, N. (2018). *Foundations of Reiki Ryoho.* Rochester: Healing Arts Press.

Penman, D. (2015). *Mindfulness for Creativity: Adapt, Create and Thrive in a Frantic World*. London: Piatkus.

Petter, F.A. (1997). *Reiki Fire.* Twin Lakes: Lotus Light Publications.

Petter, F.A. and Usui, M. (1999). *The Original Reiki Handbook of Mikao Usui.* Twin Lakes: Lotus Press.

Petter, F., Yamaguchi, T. and Hayashi, C. (2003). *The Hayashi*

Reiki Manual. Twin Lakes: Lotus Press.

Petter, F.A. (2012). *This Is Reiki.* Twin Lakes: Lotus Press.

Preece, R. (2006). *The Psychology of Buddhist Tantra.* Ithaca: Snow Lion.

Quest, P. (2002). *Reiki for Life: The Complete Guide to Reiki Practice for Levels 1, 2 & 3.* London: Piatkus.

Quest, P. (2004). Just for Today: Living with the Reiki Principles – Part 1. *Reiki News Magazine,* 3(3).

Rajkumar, N. (2014). *Why do you tell people not to do Healing? Sadhguru.* [video] Available at: https://www.youtube.com/watch?v=74G_FKQeCAY [Accessed 3 Apr. 2019].

Rajsuddhinanamongkol, P. (1997). *Advantages of Chanting and How to Practice Vipassana Meditation.* Wat Ambhavan: Suchitra Ronruen.

Reese, R. (2003). *Different Yet the Same: Kami and Shen.* [online] Robertjamesreese.com. Available at: https://robertjamesreese.com/essays/different-yet-the-same-kami-and-shen [Accessed 8 Apr. 2019].

Reid, D. (1998). *Chi-Gung: Harnessing the Power of the Universe.* 1st ed. London: Simon & Schuster.

Rinpoche, R. (2017). *Lazy Lama Looks at Loving Kindness.* Hereford: Bodhicharya Publications.

Rinpoche, S. (1992). *The Tibetan Book of Living and Dying.* London: Rider.

Rinpoche, T. (2009). *The Three Kayas.* [online] The Dharma Corner. Available at: https://dharmacorner.blogspot.com/2009/08/three-kayas.html [Accessed 18 Feb. 2020].

Rinpoche, H.E. (2013). *The Four Noble Truths.* [online] tsemrinpoche.com. Available at: https://www.tsemrinpoche.com/tsem-tulku-rinpoche/external-article/the-four-noble-truths-2?gclid=CjwKCAjwguzzBRBiEiwAgU0FT2w4htmgNfNS0-HLm57rIuhKuQlx8_dDQccx84rUQkZx6sxRMu63fhoCq_UQAvD_BwE [Accessed 26th March 2020].

Rivard, R. (n.d.). *Origin of the Reiki Attunement.* [online] The

Reiki Threshold. Available at: https://www.threshold.ca/reiki/Origin-of-the-Reiki-Attunement.html [Accessed 4 Apr. 2019].

Rivard, R. (n.d.). *Traditional Reiki Symbols.* [online] The Reiki Threshold. Available at: http://www.threshold.ca/reiki/sample/index.html [Accessed 15th Aug. 2019].

Ryu, S. (n.d.). *What Is Hotsuma Tutsae?* [online] Japanophilia. Available at: https://japanophilia.xyz/2018/06/06/hotsuma-tsutae/ [Accessed 18 Aug. 2019].

Sacredlotus.com. (n.d.). *Shen (Spirit) In Chinese Medicine.* [online] Sacred Lotus Chinese Medicine. Available at: <https://www.sacredlotus.com/go/foundations-chinese-medicine/get/shen-spirit-chinese-medicine> [Accessed 30 May 2020].

Salzberg, S. (1995). *Loving-Kindness: The Revolutionary Art of Happiness.* Boulder: Shambhala Publications Inc.

Samsen, J. and Hanson, H. (n.d.). *The Dan Tien — Three Major Energy Megalopolises of the Body.* [online] The Gathering – Metaphysical Guidebook. Available at: https://metaphysicalguidebook.wordpress.com/3-2/the-dan-tien-three-major-energy-megalopolises-of-the-body/ [Accessed 31 Mar. 2019].

Sangharakshita. (2004). *Living with Kindness: The Buddha's Teachings on Metta.* Cambridge: Windhorse Publications.

Schumacher, M. (2011). *Mandala or Mandara.* [online] A to Z Photo Dictionary Japanese Buddhist Statuary. Available at: https://www.onmarkproductions.com/html/mandala1.shtml [Accessed 22 Sep. 2019].

Segal, Z. (2016). *The Three-Minute Breathing Space Practice.* [online] Mindful Healthy Mind, Healthy Body. Available at: https://www.mindful.org/the-three-minute-breathing-space-practice/ [Accessed 4 Jun. 2020].

Seppala, E. (2014). *18 Science-Based Reasons to Try Loving-Kindness Meditation Today!* [online] Emma Seppälä, Ph.D. Available at: https://emmaseppala.com/18-science-based-reasons-try-loving-kindness-meditation-today/ [Accessed 14 Nov. 2019].

Sister Vajira, & Story, F. (1998). *Maha-parinibbana Sutta: Last Days of the Buddha*. [online] Accesstoinsight.org. Available at: https://www.accesstoinsight.org/tipitaka/dn/dn.16.1-6.vaji.html. [Accessed 8 Apr. 2020].

Skinner, J. and Bladen, S. (2018). *Practical Zen; for Health, Wealth and Mindfulness*. London: Singing Dragon.

Soundofom.com. (n.d.). *Om*. [online] Available at: http://soundofom.com/om/ [Accessed 6 Sep. 2019].

Stiene, B. and Stiene, F. (n.d.). *Reiki Energetic System*. [online] International House of Reiki. Available at: https://ihreiki.com/reiki_info/reiki_energetic_system/ [Accessed 30 Mar. 2019].

Stiene, B and Stiene, F. (2003). *The Reiki Sourcebook.* Winchester: O Books.

Stiene, B and Stiene, F. (2005). *The Japanese Art of Reiki.* Ropley: O Books.

Stiene, B. and Stiene, F. (2006). *Everything About Reiju*. [online] International House of Reiki. Available at: https://ihreiki.com/blog/everything_about_reiju/ [Accessed 5 Apr. 2019].

Stiene, B. and Stiene, F. (2008). *The Deeper Meaning of Hara*. [online] International House of Reiki. Available at: https://ihreiki.com/blog/the_deeper_meaning_of_hara/ [Accessed 4 Apr. 2019].

Stiene, F. (2015). *The Inner Heart of Reiki: Rediscovering Your True Self.* Winchester. Ayni Books.

Stiene, F. (2018). *Reiki Insights.* Winchester: Ayni Books.

The New Yoga. (n.d.). *TANTRA AND TAOISM On their Essential Nature and Relation*. [online] Available at: http://www.thenewyoga.org/tantra_and_taoism.htm [Accessed 8 Apr. 2019].

Sumedho, A. (1995). *The Mind and The Way: Buddhist Reflections on Life.* London: Rider.

Suzuki, S. (2011). *Zen Mind, Beginners Mind: Informal Talks on*

Zen Meditation and Practice. 40th ed. Boulder: Shambhala Publications, Inc.

Tantrapa, L. (2007). *Qi Dao – Tibetan Shamanic Qigong.* Author House.

Thacer1112 (2012). *Sadhguru Why One Should not do Reiki to Avoid Karma.* [video] Available at: https://www.youtube.com/watch?v=9A2RZOMqJgw [Accessed 4 Jul. 2019].

The Online Etymology Dictionary. (n.d.). *(heal v.).* [online] Available at: https://www.etymonline.com/search?q=heal [Accessed 4 Jul. 2019].

Trungpa, C. (1981). *Journey Without Goal: The Tantric Wisdom of the Buddha.* Massachusetts: Shambhala Publications Inc.

Usarzewicz, W. (2015). *Learn Reiki Meditations – Gassho and Joshin Kokyu Ho.* [online] Reikipaths. Available at: http://reikipaths.com/p/gassho-joshin-kokyu-ho/118# [Accessed 17 Apr. 2019].

Vessantara. (1998). *Meeting the Buddhas: A Guide to Buddhas, Bodhisattvas, and Tantric Deities.* Birmingham: Windhorse Publications.

Vessantara. (2005). *The Art of Meditation: The Breath.* Cambridge: Windhorse Publications.

Vennells, D. (2005). *Reiki Mastery: For Second Degree Students and Masters.* 1st ed. Ropley: O Books.

Williams, M et al., (2007). *The Mindful Way Through Depression.* New York: The Guilford Press.

Wikipedia The Free Encyclopedia. (n.d.). *Mudra.* [online] Available at: https://en.wikipedia.org/wiki/*Mudra* [Accessed 20 Apr. 2019].

Wikipedia The Free Encyclopedia. (n.d.). *Yantra.* [online) Available at: https://en.wikipedia.org/wiki/Yantra#Usage_and_meaning [Accessed 9 Feb. 2020].

Yamaguchi, T. (2007). *Light on the Origins of Reiki: A Handbook for Practicing the Original Reiki of Usui and Hayashi.* 1st ed. Twin Lakes: Lotus Press – Shangri-La.

Yogapedia.com. (n.d.). *What Is Sambhogakaya? – Definition from Yogapedia.* [online] Available at: https://www.yogapedia.com/definition/11020/Sambhogakaya [Accessed 6 Sep. 2019].

Your Dictionary (n.d.). Bodhisattva. [online] Available at: https://www.yourdictionary.com/bodhisattva [Accessed 9 Feb. 2020].

Zeidan, F., Emerson, N., Farris, S., Ray, J., Jung, Y., McHaffie, J. and Coghill, R., (2015). Mindfulness Meditation-Based Pain Relief Employs Different Neural Mechanisms Than Placebo and Sham Mindfulness Meditation-Induced Analgesia. *Journal of Neuroscience,* 35(46), pp.15307–15325.

Zhang, S. (2008). *Compare Dan Tien to Chakra?* [online] The Dao Bums: Discussions on the Way. Available at: https://www.thedaobums.com/topic/6876-compare-dan-tien-to-chakra/ [Accessed 31 Mar. 2019].

Zopa. (2011). *The Practice Called Opening the Eye.* [ebook] Portland: FPMT Inc. Available at: https://shop.fpmt.org/Prayer-to-Chenrezig-Compassionate-Eye-Looking-One-PDF_p_3137.html [Accessed 24 Aug. 2019].

AYNI
BOOKS

ALTERNATIVE HEALTH & HEALING

"Ayni" is a Quechua word meaning "reciprocity" - sharing, giving and receiving - whatever you give out comes back to you. To be in Ayni is to be in balance, harmony and right relationship with oneself and nature, of which we are all an intrinsic part. Complementary and Alternative approaches to health and well-being essentially follow a holistic model, within which one is given support and encouragement to move towards a state of balance, true health and wholeness, ultimately leading to the awareness of one's unique place in the Universal jigsaw of life - Ayni, in fact. If you have enjoyed this book, why not tell other readers by posting a review on your preferred book site.

Recent bestsellers from AYNI Books are:

Reclaiming Yourself from Binge Eating
A Step-By-Step Guide to Healing
Leora Fulvio, MFT
Win the war against binge eating, wake up each morning at peace with your body, unafraid of food and overeating.
Paperback: 978-1-78099-680-6 ebook: 978-1-78099-681-3

The Reiki Sourcebook (revised ed.)
Frans Stiene, Bronwen Stiene
A popular, comprehensive and updated manual for the Reiki novice, teacher and general reader.
Paperback: 978-1-84694-181-8 ebook: 978-1-84694-648-6

The Chakras Made Easy
Hilary H. Carter
From the successful Made Easy series, Chakras Made Easy is a practical guide to healing the seven chakras.
Paperback: 978-1-78099-515-1 ebook: 978-1-78099-516-8

The Inner Heart of Reiki
Rediscovering Your True Self
Frans Stiene
A unique journey into the inner heart of the system of Reiki, to help practitioners and teachers rediscover their True Selves.
Paperback: 978-1-78535-055-9 ebook: 978-1-78535-056-6

Middle Age Beauty
Soulful Secrets from a Former Face Model Living Botox Free in her Forties
Machel Shull
Find out how to look fabulous during middle age without plastic surgery by learning inside secrets from a former model.
Paperback: 978-1-78099-574-8 ebook: 978-1-78099-575-5

The Optimized Woman
Using Your Menstrual Cycle to Achieve Success and Fulfillment
Miranda Gray
If you want to get ahead, get a cycle! For women who want to create life-success in a female way.
Paperback: 978-1-84694-198-6

The Patient in Room Nine Says He's God
Louis Profeta
A roller coaster ride of joy, controversy, triumph and tragedy; often all on the same page.
Paperback: 978-1-84694-354-6 ebook: 978-1-78099-736-0

Re-humanizing Medicine
A Holistic Framework for Transforming Your Self, Your Practice, and the Culture of Medicine
David Raymond Kopacz
Re-humanizing medical practice for doctors, clinicians, clients, and systems.
Paperback: 978-1-78279-075-4 ebook: 978-1-78279-074-7

You Can Beat Lung Cancer Using Alternative/Integrative Interventions
Carl O. Helvie R.N., Dr.P.H.
Significantly increase your chances of long-term lung cancer survival by using holistic alternative and integrative interventions by physicians or health practitioners.
Paperback: 978-1-78099-283-9 ebook: 978-1-78099-284-6

Readers of ebooks can buy or view any of these bestsellers by clicking on the live link in the title. Most titles are published in paperback and as an ebook. Paperbacks are available in traditional bookshops. Both print and ebook formats are available online.

Find more titles and sign up to our readers' newsletter at http://www.johnhuntpublishing.com/mind-body-spirit
Follow us on Facebook at https://www.facebook.com/OBooks and Twitter at https://twitter.com/obooks